# FAITH AND THE PURSUIT OF HEALTH

## MEDICAL ANTHROPOLOGY: HEALTH, INEQUALITY, AND SOCIAL JUSTICE

Series editor: Lenore Manderson

Books in the Medical Anthropology series are concerned with social patterns of and social responses to ill health, disease, and suffering, and how social exclusion and social justice shape health and healing outcomes. The series is designed to reflect the diversity of contemporary medical anthropological research and writing, and will offer scholars a forum to publish work that showcases the theoretical sophistication, methodological soundness, and ethnographic richness of the field.

Books in the series may include studies on the organization and movement of peoples, technologies, and treatments, how inequalities pattern access to these, and how individuals, communities and states respond to various assaults on wellbeing, including from illness, disaster, and violence.

Jessica Hardin, *Faith and the Pursuit of Health: Cardiometabolic Disorders in Samoa*
Carina Heckert, *Fault Lines of Care: Gender, HIV, and Global Health in Bolivia*
Alison Heller, *Fistula Politics: Birthing Injuries and the Quest for Continence in Niger*
Joel Christian Reed, *Landscapes of Activism: Civil Society and HIV and AIDS Care in Northern Mozambique*
Beatriz M. Reyes-Foster, *Psychiatric Encounters: Madness and Modernity in Yucatan, Mexico*
Sonja van Wichelen, *Legitimating Life: Adoption in the Age of Globalization and Biotechnology*
Lesley Jo Weaver, *Sugar and Tension: Diabetes and Gender in Modern India*
Andrea Whittaker, *International Surrogacy as Disruptive Industry in Southeast Asia*

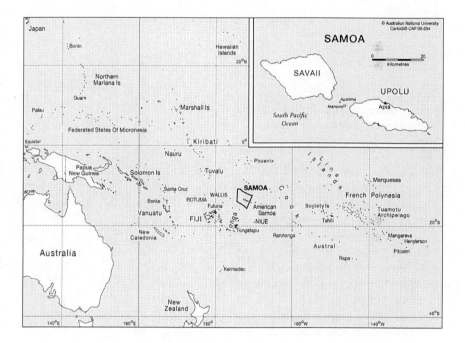

# FAITH AND THE PURSUIT OF HEALTH

## Cardiometabolic Disorders in Samoa

JESSICA HARDIN

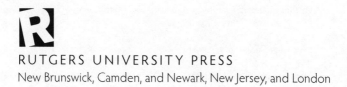

RUTGERS UNIVERSITY PRESS
New Brunswick, Camden, and Newark, New Jersey, and London

Library of Congress Cataloging-in-Publication Data

Names: Hardin, Jessica A., author.
Title: Faith and the pursuit of health : cardiometabolic disorders in Samoa /
    Jessica Hardin.
Description: New Brunswick, New Jersey : Rutgers University Press, [2018] |
    Series: Medical anthropology | Includes bibliographical references and index.
Identifiers: LCCN 2018004275| ISBN 9780813592930 (cloth : alk. paper) |
    ISBN 9780813592923 (pbk. : alk. paper) | ISBN 9780813592947 (epub) |
    ISBN 9780813592961 (Web PDF)
Subjects: LCSH: Church work with the sick—Samoa. | Church work with the
    sick—Pentecostal churches. | Cardiovascular system—Diseases. |
    Obesity—Samoa.
Classification: LCC BV4460 .H29 2018 | DDC 613.099614—dc23
LC record available at https://lccn.loc.gov/2018004275

A British Cataloging-in-Publication record for this book is available from the
British Library.

Unless otherwise indicated, all photographs copyright © Jessica Hardin

www.rutgersuniversitypress.org

Manufactured in the United States of America

For Apulu
and
Greg and George

# CONTENTS

# FOREWORD

## LENORE MANDERSON

Medical Anthropology: Health, Inequality, Social Justice is a new series from Rutgers University Press designed to capture the diversity of contemporary medical anthropological research and writing. The beauty of ethnography is its capacity, through storytelling, to make sense of suffering as a social experience, and to set it in context. Central to our focus in this series on health, illness, and social justice, therefore, is the way in which social structures and ideologies shape the likelihood and impact of infections, injuries, bodily ruptures and disease, chronic conditions and disability, treatment and care, social repair, and death.

The brief for this series is broad. The books are concerned with health and illness, healing practices and access to care, but the authors illustrate too the importance of context—of geography, physical condition, service availability, and income. Health and illness are social facts; the circumstances of the maintenance and loss of health are always and everywhere shaped by structural, global, and local relations. Society, culture, economy, and political organization as much as ecology shape the variance of illness, disability, and disadvantage. But as medical anthropologists have long illustrated, the relationships of social context and health status are complex. In addressing these questions, the authors in this series showcase the theoretical sophistication, methodological rigor, and empirical richness of the field, while expanding a map of illness and social and institutional life to illustrate the effects of material conditions and social meanings in troubling and surprising ways.

The books in the series move across social circumstances, health conditions, and geography, and their intersections and interactions, to demonstrate how individuals, communities, and states manage assaults on well-being. The books reflect medical anthropology as a constantly changing field of scholarship, drawing on research diversely in residential and virtual communities, clinics and laboratories, in emergency care and public health settings, with service providers, individual healers and households, with social bodies, human bodies, and biologies. While medical anthropology once concentrated on systems of healing, particular diseases, and embodied experiences, today the field has expanded to include environmental disaster and war, science, technology and faith, gender-based violence, and forced migration. Curiosity about the body and its vicissitudes remains a pivot for our work, but our concerns are with the location of bodies in social life, and with how social structures, temporal imperatives, and shifting exigencies shape life courses. This dynamic field reflects an ethics of the discipline to address these pressing issues of our time.

Globalization has contributed to and adds to the complexity of influences on health outcomes; it (re)produces social and economic relations that institutionalize poverty, unequal conditions of everyday life and work, and environments in which diseases increase or subside. Globalization patterns the movement and relations of peoples, technologies and knowledge, programs and treatments; it shapes differences in health experience and outcomes across space; it informs and amplifies inequalities at individual and country levels. Global forces and local inequalities compound and constantly load on individuals to impact on their physical and mental health, and on their households and communities. At the same time, as the subtitle of this series indicates, we are concerned with questions of social exclusion and inclusion, social justice and repair, again both globally and in local settings. The books will challenge readers to reflect not only on sickness and suffering, deficit, and despair, but also on resistance and restitution—on how people respond to injustices and evade the fault lines that might seem to predetermine life outcomes. While not all of the books take this direction, the aim is to widen the frame within which we conceptualize embodiment and suffering.

In *Faith and the Pursuit of Health*, Jessica Hardin describes the impact of globalization on diet and health on Samoans. From the mid-twentieth century, wage labor and urbanization in much of the Pacific precipitated dietary change, with traditional island foods such as fresh fish, meat, and local fruits and vegetables steadily displaced by cheaper imported foods including rice, sugar, flour, canned meats and fish, sugar-sweetened beverages, and beer. The consequence of this, with increased sedentary occupations, was rising rates of obesity and related cardiometabolic disorders—type II diabetes, hypertension, and heart disease. By the late 1970s, Pacific Island populations were emblematic of the interactions of poverty, poor food choice, and food preferences, of genetic factors that might impact metabolic change, and of local values related to body size and wealth (see, among many publications, Nanditha et al. 2016; Zimmet 1979). Forty years later, Pacific populations continue to experience poor nutrition, little exercise, and high rates of obesity and associated disease.

Against this epidemiological context and the social determinants that have fueled it, Jessica Hardin takes a fresh stance on fat, health, and fitness and, in so doing, brings together the fields of medical anthropology and the anthropology of religion. Drawing on her close everyday engagement with Samoan families and the churches to which they belong, Hardin describes how poverty, unemployment, and the obligations of gender, kinship, and church membership shape food choice and patterns of consumption; in the context of local expectations of reciprocity, commensality, and gifts, there is considerable contradiction and ambivalence in health talk about food, fat, and fitness. As Hardin illustrates, Pentecostal church membership provides many people with ways to negotiate these pressures. New forms of social support and new perspectives on individual and community obligations are incorporated into people's understandings of disease causality, and impact on the possibilities available to them of health practices such as diet, exercise, and weight loss. Pentecostal understandings shed light on how people navigate social change, and offer them new ways to enhance their own and others' health. Unexpectedly, in attributing responsibility for their health problems and social circumstances to God, Pentecostal Samoans find a measure of agency not otherwise afforded in daily life, and thus faith and church membership support their efforts to improve their health.

# NOTE ON PRONUNCIATION

Samoan terms used in the body of this book follow contemporary Samoan orthographic conventions. The letter "g" is used to represent the velar nasal and is pronounced like an English "ng." The glottal stop is represented by an apostrophe and is pronounced like the missing consonant in the cockney pronunciation of "bottle" (bo'le). The long vowel is characterized by a macron over the vowel (e.g., ā) and indicates a lengthened articulation of the vowel. In modern Samoan, writing the glottal stop and macron is often omitted from the written representation of a word, but they are always pronounced.

# FAITH AND THE PURSUIT OF HEALTH

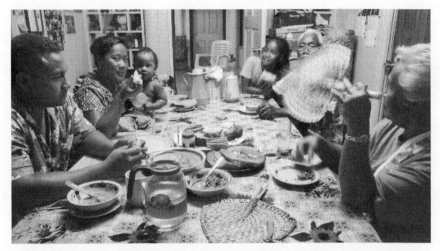

FIGURE 1 The rain hit the roof, reverberating a tinny sound throughout the house. We ate light food on nights like tonight, nights where it was both muggy and cool, the air heavy with rain and all things a little moist from the stretch of rainy days that proceeded. We drank milky black tea that was heavy from sugar, to keep warm and fend off sickness. Eating light meant sandwiches with tinned fish or pisūpo, soup—a broth of chicken and kapisi, leafy greens that the youngest son grew in the garden behind the house. We also ate fa'i Samoa, that is, Samoan bananas. They are fat; that's why they are called fa'i Samoa. These are the bananas you eat with family, not guests. The good ones are fa'i pālagi; they are skinny like white people.

# 1 · SALVATION AND METABOLISM

To arrive at Lonise's office, you must first circle through the flea market, past clothing and tourist vendors, with the smells of fish and chips and bus exhaust wafting through the air. I was encouraged to contact Lonise, a forty-nine-year-old Pentecostal business executive, because she had just given a talk about faith and health at a women's leadership conference. Her offices were on the sixth floor of one of the tallest buildings in Samoa, and when I arrived at the front desk and asked to see her, the receptionist, quite skeptical of my request, had to confirm my appointment with Lonise's two executive assistants.[1] Once I was cleared, the receptionist quickly escorted me to her office and respectfully served me a glass of cold water on a tray. At the time, I didn't realize that part of the reason it took so much effort to reach Lonise was because the staff treated Lonise as their "spiritual mum," a respected elder who deserved care, protection, and attention.

Gazing out onto the twinkling Pacific Ocean, Lonise said, "God is good, no?" After introducing myself again (we had only spoken on the phone), she said, "I am so happy to talk with you about all the blessings Father has provided." I started by asking Lonise about the conference. "Basically, I talked to working women about their spiritual health, telling them that the person is spirit first. We are made of three parts: spirit, body, and soul. But, we are first and foremost spirit. If you believe the Bible, it says you have eternal life, but it is actually only the spirit that lives forever." The spirit, body, and soul, however, "are tied tightly together," making neglect in one area register in another. While the body is only temporary material (i.e., it "dies, but the soul lives"), it is still affected by the state of the spirit.

Excited to share more, Lonise went on to explain that healing was the everyday practice of keeping these parts "balanced." She explained, as I heard from many others, that "healing is the children's bread. It's supposed to be sustenance. That is your subsistence diet. Even the dogs live off the crumbs that fall off the table." I was intrigued by the idea that healing was a kind of food, particularly because it countered popular stereotypes of faith healing as instantaneous and miraculous—the image of a woman free of crutches comes to mind. Instead, Lonise articulated what I came to learn from many: healing was an everyday necessity that could change the state of the body while also maintaining health. Given the epidemiological profile of Samoa, where rates of chronic cardiometabolic disorders including diabetes, hypertension, heart disease, and kidney disease have all rapidly increased since the 1950s—all in association with dietary change, Lonise's food analogy was even more provocative.[2]

Lonise's ideas about healing were informed by her own experience with illness. "You see, I was very sick," she said, "that's when I found the Lord." When Lonise was hospitalized for what she would learn was a stroke, she also learned she had *toto maualuga* (high blood pressure). She remembered this vividly, as this was the time she was born again. "Some friends came over and prayed over me," she said. "We did the prayer of salvation. I accepted Jesus in myself." When I asked her what she understood caused her illness, Lonise responded by talking about her church affiliation. "In those days, I was EFKS" (*Ekalesia Faapotopotoga Kerisiano Samoa*, Congregational Church of Samoa).[3] Her family and church were deeply entwined. Her parents were elders in the church and they had been attending that church for many generations—as many as Lonise could remember. This was one more reason she traveled over an hour each Sunday to attend services. "I would go to church and pray, but I never actually felt His presence. I never came to know Him. I never felt an intimacy with the Lord, until I accepted Jesus in my heart." Lonise articulated a common Pentecostal experience: mainstream Christianity did not provide opportunities to experience intimacy with God, and only after being born again could she feel close and intimately familiar with God. Lonise's story, however, is also unique to this context because she yoked together her conversion with "control" of her high blood pressure.

Lonise was elegant and well educated; her *puletasi* (Samoan-made women's clothing) were well fitted and made from Samoan boutique-designed fabrics. These puletasi, her overseas education, her job as an executive, and her residence in Apia, the capital, and only city in Samoa, indicated wealth, yet Lonise was "stressed and worried about money all the time." Discussions of "stress" and "worry" about money were the norm among the people with whom I talked from across religious, economic, and geographic backgrounds. In part, this reflected the intensity of commitment to family in Samoa, which was often expressed through gifts. Contributing cash, providing food and meals, and sharing textile valuables were measures of commitment to family (see also Addo 2013, for examples from Tonga). In Samoa, giving takes two primary forms: *fa'alavelave* (ritual exchange events) and church offerings. Fa'alavelave are large-scale ritual exchange events organized around major life events like weddings and funerals. Church offerings to pastors and their families are also a measure of family commitment, as churches are embedded within villages and family histories are interwoven with church histories. Giving to church is intense, and in addition to multiple annual giving campaigns, people are expected to give weekly. Both forms of giving are public demonstrations of family solidarity, while also generating daily expressions of stress and unhappiness (see also Gershon 2000, 2006).

Lonise felt that weekly church contributions made participation "more about competition than about knowing Jesus." She connected this disassociated feeling from church as a disassociated feeling with her family, leading her to "party," which was a way to talk about drinking, smoking, and not spending time with her kids, revealing a broader Pentecostal moral concern with the consumption of alcohol, cigarettes, and marijuana (see Brusco 1995; Cole 2012; Everett and Ramirez 2015). Combining health promotion knowledge about the risks of drinking and smoking with a Christian moralization of indulgence, Lonise and others connected multiple forms of moral consumption with the risks of cardiometabolic disorders. "I was depressed," she told me, and she felt "low, like low energy all the time." With conversion, Lonise began to link these embodied experiences with being unsaved, and she felt that her chronic sickness reflected her chronic distance from God. Church, in her view, was more a source of stress than of health. I asked her how her health differed now than a few years earlier. She said, "I was saved":

> You see things—the big picture now as opposed to seeing things as all about me. That's why I would get flustered and stressed, but it's not all about us. You know, it's a perspective, [conversion] puts things in their right perspective. Because when you see when everything is to do with you, all things are magnified. Your problems that seem big could actually be mole hills. But we turn them into mountains because you think it is all about you and your little life. When you see things in the big picture and you see God, there is an Almighty God there who can help you. Your problems are small by comparison. That's the reality.

Conversion helped Lonise reframe her understanding of the daily stresses that she thought caused her sickness. By turning to God, Lonise came to see these daily stresses as distractions from developing a closeness with God, and these distractions damaged her health. While Christianity is a religion ideologically focused on individual salvation—as the above passage makes clear, Lonise also found conversion helped her to understand herself in relation to others. By changing her perspective, she felt she could stay "peaceful even though she still had many problems with [her] family." In this way, Pentecostal Christianity socialized the body, helping believers to see the body, and sickness or health, as indicators of suffering or faith. When Pentecostals such as Lonise interpreted bodily sensations like stress or symptoms like lethargy as indicative of the health of social relationships, they integrated sociality into the fabric of their bodies. In turn, managing the body and the spirit were articulations of each other, despite a Christian ideology that devalues the body as "mere flesh."

In the current epidemiological moment, the body reveals the state of relationships through a temporality of chronicity—that is, the on-going, potentially escalating, quality of living with illness when a return to a "before" diagnosis is impossible (Manderson and Smith-Morris 2010; see also Manderson and Warren 2016). Lonise brought this kind of temporality forward when she said that conversion "is not a single moment," but "becoming a Christian is like changing your lifestyle; it's an everyday thing." From her perspective, her healing not only eradicated disease, but also affected her everyday practices, including "tending to my health, seeing the doctor," and "praying for strength" to deal with the stresses of church and family. Lonise remembered "changing from a baby Christian to a mature Christian" as a time of simultaneous embodied changes. As she began to lose weight, and her doctors reported her blood pressure was under control, she also began to feel "the fire of the Holy Spirit."[4] She used the term "lifestyle" to explain how her spiritual development precipitated her cardiometabolic health, with her conversion triggered by the event of her stroke. Pentecostal moral concerns with health linked cardiometabolic and emotional health with a broad range of consumptive practices—from eating to smoking, drinking, and lack of sleep. This practical framing of everyday practices as (im)moral health behaviors was one way that many Pentecostals began to think about their health as a matter of faith. Healing was thus a practical process of conversion and medical interventions where medicine was effective only because conversion predated interventions.

Lonise began to measure her development as a Christian in terms of her health changes, but other changes also started at this time. She started attending Pentecostal services during the week, and her husband also converted. Within a year, she stopped attending her family church, and this lessened her experiences of financial pressure. Like so many Samoans I encountered, she felt "free and peaceful" in her new Pentecostal church because she was no longer obligated to give money; she had freedom to worship charismatically, she chose how to give to the church, and she could "claim healing as [her] right." Healing, giving, and worship were sutured together as a source of wellness that shaped Lonise's life story. Her conversion, rather than her stroke, punctuated her life story in ways that encouraged her to become reflective and critical of her relationships, showing how some Pentecostals came to understand individual health as a proxy for an individual relatedness.

Lonise introduced me to a narrative I found to be common in Samoa. Conversion prompted by suffering from a cardiometabolic illness event encouraged sick persons to link the state of their relationships with their illnesses, and only faith could change this. As I began listening for similar logics in rituals, prayer groups, and sermons, I came to see that etiologies were scalable. In other words, while individual experiences of sickness reflected unequal access to cash, food, and even prestige, population-wide shifts in weight and disease were evidence of broader social and economic changes. Cardiometabolic disorders were both sickness and metaphor that helped people understand how macro changes in the economy—shifted demands for cash and the foods that people ate—impacted the self through their relationships to others. This was not a critique of westernized diets or fatty foods, but instead a critique of the ways that cash inequalities made relationships between people and with God challenging. Faith revealed this critical juncture as Pentecostal frameworks positioned the body as a site for knowing God, precisely because faith ideologies encouraged people to see how their relationships shaped interior states in ways that generated health or sickness.

Healing therefore could be directed at individuals and collectives, as Lonise understood. She started a prayer group in her workplace and became a "spiritual mum" in the office. After a few meetings, Lonise invited me to join, so for nearly a year, I sat with her and her work colleagues during their lunch hour as they prayed about everything from office relationships to corruption in the government. The group worked with deliverance and healing methods to define and identify sources of suffering and by naming the source; they aimed to command "the departure of negative emotion and behavior" (Csordas 1994, 166).[5] The group of up to fifteen met in the office conference room, seated in plush chairs tightly arranged around a slick conference table (see also Hardin 2016c). One afternoon during the intercession period (when each member individually prayed in various ways, from prostration to speaking in tongues to quiet reflection), Lagi, the office manager, grabbed her arms and massaged her joints, elbows, fingers, ankles, and knees. Amidst a cacophony of prayers, Lagi switched from glossolalia to praying in a mixture of Samoan and English, saying, "I deliver you Samoa" from the spirits of *suka* (diabetes) and *kipi* (amputations). Lagi paced the room with closed eyes, her voice raised and breathy. Finally, she said, "Samoa, you are healed." With that she sat down, quiet and tired. Later, when the group discussed the messages they had received from the Holy Spirit, Lonise shared that recently she had also felt pain in her joints, which she interpreted as a message from the Holy Spirit that "confirmed" Lagi's message. The group was constantly redefining its "mission" as a prayer group, so that when two or more members "received" related messages, they interpreted this confluence as "confirmation." The pain was shared and, therefore, understood as a "message" that the group should continue to intercede against cardiometabolic disorders. When it was Lagi's turn to share, she explained that "so many people have diabetes and amputations that it must be the devil." She continued: "Some people in our group have these spirits but have been delivered when they accepted Jesus Christ. We must bring this message to Samoa and do our mission."

These stories of Lonise and Lagi illustrate how conversion and cardiometabolic health were linked. Salvation promised healing of the individual as a step toward healing communities, showing how even individualistic practices of healing were social.[6] In turn, healing was an idiom through which newly born-again Christians came to stitch together individualist endeavors—salvation, metabolism—with the social context of those endeavors. Healing practices provided a straightforward way to transform individual bodies while impacting the broader community, making evident the problems of the collective in the bodies of individual Christians. I refer to this as *embodied critique*. This allows me to describe how Pentecostals interpret bodily evidence according to a cardiometabolic logic that explained the ups and downs of glucose, weight, or blood pressure as reflections of fluctuations in faith, linking both bodily symptoms and faith to the perils of being a good Christian in a changing social and economic world. When Lonise redirected her resources and strived to develop closeness with God, she experienced a reduction in stress. Faith helped her to change aspects of her life that she felt affected her health. In her case, cardiometabolic health was derived from her faith. She brought that godly state into being through her actions; God didn't instantly restore cardiometabolic balance. She had to work to change her environment and behaviors, which was difficult, but when framed through the lens of faith, "everything is possible," she would say. In turn, she redirected her responsibility for her health as responsibility to God to create the Kingdom of God on Earth—an expression of salvation. This is not a subtle rehearsing of the Christian individual or the biomedical citizen; instead, Pentecostal perspectives show how invisible metrics and mundane symptoms of cardiometabolic disorders—like headaches, dizziness, and sores—signified the state of relationships, which ultimately reverberated through the body metabolically. In this way, Christian and chronic illness identities were both states of *becoming* that made spiritual self-work and cardiometabolic self-care virtuous.

## CARDIOMETABOLIC DISORDERS AS A CHRISTIAN PROBLEM

Today, Samoa regularly appears on "top fattest nation" lists in global media, making Samoa famous for its disease profile (for examples, see Jacobs 2016; Swanson 2015). Some Samoans see recent work by medical and biocultural anthropologists on high levels of obesity as exoticizing Samoan culture to the outside world. Representations of the "noncommunicable disease epidemic" are mobilized by global organizations such as the World Health Organization and the Food and Agriculture Organization, dominated by foreign voices and interests. A quick Internet search with the words "obesity" and "Samoa" returns countless links to public health research, news reporting on "the epidemic," and a slew of images of brown, obese bodies—often "headless fatties"—and fatty meats (Cooper 2007). Samoa also made international headlines when Samoa Air began charging passengers by their weight instead of a standard fare.

As this cartoon makes clear, fat is associated with primitiveness, where Polynesians are unable to adapt to this new environment filled with fatty, salty, and highly processed foods. The primitiveness is defined not only by the fact that their

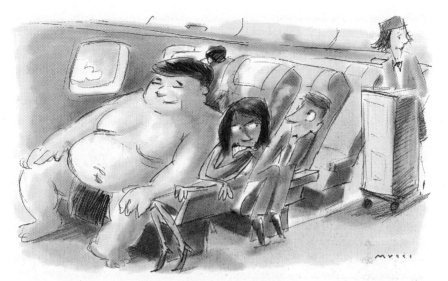

FIGURE 2 Illustrated by Michael Mucci. First appeared in the *Sydney Morning Herald*, January 13, 2012.

bodies do not fit within modern infrastructures, like airplanes, but that they also do not understand the need for change in diet and lifestyle. These primitive bodies are represented as a burden, which the red-faced passenger makes clear. The obesity epidemic is thus represented as specifically Polynesian, which Samoan health professionals upheld in their views that *fa'asamoa* (Samoan culture, the Samoan way) was both the cause and the solution to this so-called epidemic. On the one hand, health professionals argued that Samoan "mentalities" linking fatness with health and large portions with satiety, and deprioritized healthcare, were the source of the rapid rise in cardiometabolic disorders, articulating the misfit as depicted in the cartoon (Hardin 2015a). On the other hand, health practitioners valued the culture of care for elders and saw that the church and land were essential components to any successful intervention. Obesity research, both globally and locally, therefore contributes to the circulation of images and ideas about Pacific Islander obesity, which, in turn, can further stigmatize fatness as articulated both locally and globally.

Bodies of Samoans, and Pacific Islanders more generally, have become synonymous with obesity.[7] Research in the Samoan islands and the diaspora has come to be used as "a rough but meaningful gradient of exposure to the influences of modern life" (Brewis 2011, 50). On this gradient, Samoa represents the "least modernized," followed by American Samoa and then diaspora centers in the United States, New Zealand, and Australia. Because of this research history and the ways resources flow as a result of it (including through research grants, volunteer organizations, and a medical school), "new medical missionaries" seem to flock to

Samoa in greater numbers each year to examine issues associated with cardiometabolic disorders (Panosian and Coates 2006). Or at least Samoan health officials intimated that this was how it felt. This steady flow of research interest, with ranging professionalism and purpose, made research both a common-sense endeavor and one that funneled data about fat outward for global evaluation.

This context of globally mediated representations of Pacific fatness and the influx of health promotion activities has made most Samoans knowledgeable of population-wide rates of cardiometabolic disorders. I first learned this when I began preliminary fieldwork on Oahu, Hawai'i. Samoans I encountered there were quick to say things like, "We love our food; Samoan people love to eat" and "Samoan people are lazy; we just want to eat the easy, fatty foods." Interview after interview, and in casual conversations, I heard people reiterate the relationship between diet and sickness. These responses iterated official accounts—that is, "conventional teachings from health promotion" (Garro 2010, 472). However, the more time I spent with people, particularly in church, the more nuanced people's answers became about why Samoans get sick, and why healing was so difficult.[8]

One afternoon in Waipahu, Hawai'i, while sitting in an Assemblies of God church parking lot—a place that also served as a community space for hanging out, cooking, or dance practice, Faga, a church elder, helped me understand cardiometabolic etiologies that moved beyond these official accounts. While living in Hawai'i, Faga's husband had died because of complications from diabetes. She thought he was sick because he was storing taro he carried from Samoa in his house, stockpiling it, and not giving it away. Faga felt her husband needed to "be delivered from the spirit of greed," and she felt he was sick as a result. Others also associated gluttony and avarice with illness and talked about fasting as a way of achieving closeness with God; this resulted in them being able to change their diet in ways that affected their health, even if they were not explicitly abstaining from food for health reasons (Hardin 2013). Connecting sickness with the inappropriate social uses of food demonstrates that the value of food lies beyond its nutritional qualities. Across Oceania, ethnography tells us of places where giving food as gifts is a form of competition, a way to shame opponents through the presentation of food abundance (Young 1971; Kahn and Sexton 1988; Manderson 1986; Pollock 1992; Whitehead 2000; Kahn 1986).[9] In Samoa, people struggle with reducing food intake in a context where consumption of food is both a way to recognize the generosity and status of others, while creating one's own status as a receiver of food gifts (see Rosen, DePue, and McGarvey 2008). Health, similar to how native Hawaiians conceptualize it, revolves around the ability to eat and prepare cultural foods not only because they are satisfying, but also because they affirm connections between land and ancestors (McMullin 2005, 815). This project builds on these approaches because they show that food, and fat, mediate the body in ways that are deeply spiritual—food and fat connect people and ancestors through time because foods are derived from lands that families cultivate over generations.[10]

Biomedical and public health approaches to cardiometabolic disorders have tended to reduce risk to individual responsibility—that is, reduce food consumption and increase physical activity. In contrast, drawing attention to the relationship between the social world and the spirit—what I call *spiritual etiologies*—brings into focus the often multiple and flexible etiologies derived from the basic logic that environments and relationships permeate the body in ways that create sickness and health. My analysis of the experience of cardiometabolic disorders among Samoan Pentecostals is aided by the synergies of approaches between medical anthropology and the anthropology of healing and individualization in medical anthropology and the anthropology of Christianity.

Medical anthropologists have identified and studied how the medicalization of fat—that is, the process of converting the problem of weight into a medical problem—erases how that context shapes the emergence and experience of fatness and related disorders.[11] When social and economic contexts are obscured, medical problems become the responsibility of the individual not only to heal, but also to prevent illness and manage the body. Similarly, around the world, Christianity emphasizes individuality and values interiority (Keane 1997a). Christians exert a great deal of effort to create intimacy with God, which is represented as "self-generating, self-authorizing" (Handman 2015, 14). This focus on the individual subject is further compounded by the ways that neoliberal ideologies, which also individualize risk, often accompany the growth of Pentecostalism. Scholars argue that there has been an "'institutional deficit" that has resulted in people having "fewer and fewer ways to sustain spaces in which social relations can be organized by nonmarket logics to meet nonmarket goals" (Robbins 2009, 55). As a result, Pentecostal churches have prospered when other forms of institutional, state, and social support have dwindled. These synergies reveal multiple ways that ideologies of individuality propagate globally despite the fact that cardiometabolic disorders are deeply shaped by the social, economic, and ecological context.

In Samoa, across denomination and geography, people talked about cardiometabolic disorders as problems of money and markets (Hardin and Kwauk 2015). At the individual level, I heard that Samoans couldn't "afford" to purchase "healthy foods" and, at the population level, that the cost of food reflected free-market logics increasingly guiding Samoa's trade policy (Snowdon and Thow 2013; Seiden et al. 2012). In this context, healing cardiometabolic disorders was a deeply social problem, yet clinics tended to treat these disorders individually—as conditions that could be controlled or prevented through diet, exercise, and medication (compare with Yates-Doerr 2012a). As I show in this book, Pentecostalism provided multiple ways for people to see how their sicknesses were caused by social and economic problems. Pentecostal healing highlighted the limits of biomedical explanations of cardiometabolic suffering (i.e., change your diet, exercise, take your medications) by emphasizing, instead, the limitless potential of God to change the social conditions under which disease emerged. When Pentecostals talked about food, fat, and fitness, they created an understanding of the body as a mediator between social and biological determinants of health, while faith created a pathway for God to heal.

The medicalization of fat has a long history, dating particularly from the creation of a now highly contested measure, body mass index (BMI).[12] In the United States, the medicalization of fat has been so naturalized that, for most Americans, it is difficult to imagine alternative frameworks for understanding excess weight (Saguy 2013; Greenhalgh 2015). "No longer are chunky and fat people merely 'lazy,'" writes Susan Greenhalgh. "In the current discourse, they are also biologically defective; chronically ill; at risk of yet other obesity-related diseases; and in need of ongoing medical treatment" (2015, 6). These American ideas about fat are founded on the premise that the body is controlled by the individual, and so, if an individual exerts enough willpower, the body can be changed (Bordo 1993; Bell, McNaughton, and Salmon 2011). This ideology persists despite an emerging political ecology of obesity that shows how cardiometabolic disorders and obesity disproportionately affect communities of color, including indigenous populations in the United States and around the world, and poor communities everywhere (Popkin, Adair, and Ng 2012; for a summary of these global trends, see Brewis 2011, 31–32; NCD Risk Factor Collaboration 2016; Guthman 2011).

Instead of blaming individuals for weight, my interlocutors talked about not being able to afford healthy foods, for example, as a major barrier to losing weight. When they articulated this causal connection, they transformed the problem of food, fat, and fitness into a problem of faith. The problem was no longer a barrier when articulated as a problem of Christian practice—the problem was one of developing an imitate relationship with God as a means of transforming self and community. As a result, healing transformed individual responsibility into social responsibility by shifting from the register of biomedicine to the register of Christianity. Through Pentecostal healing, my interlocutors came to identify their source of suffering in the social world where relationships with humans and non-human others, including Jesus, the Holy Spirit, and evil spirits, penetrated the body.[13] Healing cardiometabolic disorders required the person to look to the context of the emergence of the illness. What was the source of the stress? What obligations were causing suffering? Bringing together these distinct anthropological ways of approaching illness shows the creative ways that structural limitations and social determinants of health were negotiated by those living with cardiometabolic disorders. They did so by embodied critique, that is, by grounding their critiques of social change in the body, and by thinking about faith through the temporality of chronicity.

## Embodied Critique

When Lonise felt her stroke was caused by stress or Lagi linked being "unsaved" with amputations, they created spiritual etiologies that tied embodied experience to relationships and symptoms to spiritual states. These etiologies suggested a critique that followed a cardiometabolic logic—the state of the spirit was knowable through metabolic evidence in the body. Shortness of breath, fat, and headaches were symptoms that could be discerned through a matrix of sociality pointing to imbalances in social relationships—with human, divine, and evil others. Courtney Handman observes that Christianity is a practice of critique where "denominational life" is a "comparative project, an unending process of Christian critique" of other people and groups (2015, 2; see also Bielo 2011). In other words, schism and denominational politics are not aberrations in Christian practice, but are characteristic of it. Critique, then, is "unavoidably *social* theory," where discerning the "social field is an essential part of Christian becoming" (emphasis original, Handman 2015, 14–15). *Faith and the Pursuit of Health* shows how this process of becoming is an embodied process and, in the context of epidemiological transformation, unfolds following a metabolic logic. This is possible because of the Christian approach to the body where bodily knowledge provides information about the world that locates an individual within a community. If metabolism suggests an embodied process of chemically converting food to "energy and body matter," embodied critique suggests that this chemical process is paralleled in the spirit (Landecker 2011, 167). The body's experiences and information garnered from the body (e.g., glucose levels, weight, hunger, dizziness) thus reveal the quality of one's relationships. We come to know our own communities through our bodies.

Metabolism is a modern metaphor for understanding the body as a mediating site (see Solomon 2016). Anthropologists have shown in other ethnographic contexts how the body, as a biological entity, is shaped by metaphor and have illustrated how these metaphors tend to naturalize cultural norms. In the United States, for example, Emily Martin (1987) described how biomedicine drew from metaphors of industrialism to understand women's bodies, with women's reproductive physiology represented as machinery and the birthing mother as a laborer. Elsewhere she describes how medical textbook accounts of reproductive biology replicate stereotypes of male and female through their renderings of egg and sperm, showing that "female biological processes are less worthy than their male counterparts" (Martin 1991, 485–486). Similarly, metabolism provides Samoan Pentecostals with a heuristic to understand how social environments shape individual bodies, whereby the cardiometabolic body is what Hannah Landecker calls a "dynamic web" creating an "iteratively generated interface" between body, spirit, and community (2011, 496, 499). Perhaps not surprising then, I often heard statements like "I felt my sugar rise" as a way to explain the effects of anger, depression, or stress on the body (see also Held et al. 2009). In other ethnographic contexts, "control" is a metaphor that implies measuring the state of the body with precision—eating right, exercising, taking medications (Naemiratch and Manderson 2006; Mol 2009; Warren et al. 2013). In Samoa, rises and falls in *suka* (blood sugar) or *toto* (blood, short for toto maualuga, high blood pressure) indicate changes in the cardiometabolic body that mirrored ambivalences about relationships. Metabolism is also invisible—one cannot see metabolism in or on the body. Yet health is dependent on managing a process that, without access to everyday measurement technologies like scales or glucometers, Samoans need other ways to make tangible this interior dynamism. In Pentecostal Christianity, an intimate God provided spiritual and discursive tools to make one's bodily interior knowable and actionable.

Metabolism was a compelling framework to understand subtle changes in the body because Samoan epistemologies of power link high-status fat bodies with sacred generation and abundant resources (Shore 1989). In Oceania, broadly speaking, the body is a community project, whereby fatness indicates community care and wealth (Becker 1995; Pollock 1995, 2011). The truism that Polynesians "think big is beautiful" is rooted in this linkage. Powerful community leaders exhibit their generative potential through their large bodies, which as a value, extends both to food and fitness. Food abundance indicates the ability to mobilize deep social networks, while stillness is the embodiment of dignity and indicates the ability to be served, further entrenching fatness as a material expression of power—both indicating wealth in food resources and people (see also Young 1971).

Christianity, however, is a religion built around ambivalence toward the body,[14] which counters indigenous Samoan approaches to the body as a source of sacred connection. With this ambivalence comes the idea that "wisdom" should be "accredited to those who claim that materiality represents the merely apparent behind that which lies that which is real" (Miller 2005, 1). This opposition between material and immaterial is an ideological dichotomy built into most religions that "dominate recorded history" where "the aim of life is to transcend the apparently obvious . . . the body as the core of our sensuous existence" (Miller 2005, 1). In contemporary Samoa, the body is both a deeply reliable source of information—as fat reveals social embeddedness—and site of temptation—reflecting Christian notions of sin. Metabolism provides a way to understand how the body feels, where health becomes evidence of transcendence and sickness becomes a symptom of distance from God.

Yet, for the people with whom I worked, healing was fleeting and it was only sustainable in relation to one's faith, which was constantly tested. In other words, faith was not constant, nor was health. Metabolism was a useful way to materially ground the changing nature of faith. In this light, the cardiometabolic body was a sensitive system that mediated social, affective, and spiritual dimensions—rendering visible that which is invisible (i.e., blood glucose levels, blood pressure). Faith "believes before seeing," my interlocutors would often say. Food, fat, and fitness were, therefore, potent symbols for understanding how the distribution of wealth affects the body—particularly because these material substances and states changed over time. This focus on the interconnections between health and wealth reflect prosperity theologies common in Pentecostal churches around the globe (Maxwell 1998; Coleman 2000). These prosperity ideas suggest that through tithes (and other gifts, sometimes referred to as "seeds" that can be "harvested") and positive speech, "believers work to integrate themselves into a heavenly economy of superabundance" (Haynes 2012, 124; 2017; Hasu 2006; Wiegele 2005). Food, fat, and fitness became "critical Christian resources" to actualize this kind of economy, allowing Samoan Pentecostals to reflect on barriers to individual immediacy with God (Handman 2015, 16). In other places around the world, Christians tend to focus on the ways that ritual or hymnals, for example, hinder individual transcendence (Engelke 2007; Meyer 2011). In Samoa, Pentecostals were concerned with the ways that hierarchy and leaders impeded direct connection to God, which made food as well as fat and fitness "good to think" with about distance from or closeness to God (Levi-Strauss 1962).[15] These critical resources were particularly illustrative because food, fat, and fitness are ordinary Samoan symbols used to exert power. However, in the context of rising rates of cardiometabolic disorders and a population-wide change in body weight, the ways fat can be linked to wellness was difficult to discern (see Yates-Doerr 2015). In everyday life, Samoans must ask themselves: How can bigger bodies exhibit strength and sacredness when fat and food abundance are also sources of sickness? What is the meaning of fat when it is no longer reserved for community leaders but is increasingly evenly distributed across the population—rich and poor, titled and untitled? As a simple example, a former mainline and now Pentecostal pastor explained to me that "the [mainline] pastors and their wives are the worst. They are the ones filling the beds at the dialysis center, and the waiting room at the diabetes clinic is filled with them too." This notion that pastors and their wives were the "worst" begged the question: If fatness can be understood as a manifestation of sacredness, why were pastors and their wives sick? Quite simply, cardiometabolic disorders raised questions about how to interpret the body when the materials that create and sustain it had changed.

Another example illuminates how questions like these were answered. Sometimes Pentecostals used the language of "blocking" to describe how pastors were recipients of myriad gifts, often described as "the best" of congregants' labor, while congregants received little in return. Mainline pastors were thought to stand at the top of a hierarchy of blessings, acting as mediators between God and community. When families gave gifts to the pastors, it was with the expectation that blessings would return, sometimes in different forms. Yet congregants felt that pastors often collected wealth in ways that did not generate blessings for the community—that is, wealth did not return to the community. When people reported that pastors were "the fattest" or "the sickest," they suggested that health and disease were indicators of how one used wealth, drawing attention to wealth that did not circulate. Embodied critique brings into focus that body size alone was insufficient to make fat meaningful. Fat derived its meaning through the process of *becoming*. Pastors' bodies were particularly effective symbols for making these kinds of determinations: Did the pastor selfishly hoard his congregants' gifts? Or did the pastor reciprocate? Was his fat a sign of his laziness or his industriousness? Looking to body size alone could not answer these questions, but Pentecostal Christianity could provide a prism through which to look at fat as a social process.

### The Chronicity of Faith

Samoan Pentecostals talked about healing as a "perfect gift" from God, meaning miracles were possible but largely dependent on the faith of the particular person seeking healing. Yet, chronic cardiometabolic illness persisted despite the faithful efforts of Christians. Diabetes never went away, even if the disease was "under control" (for a discussion of "control," see Broom and Whittaker 2004). This posed an ontological break for many Pentecostals—healing was perfectly and universally possible, yet some diseases were incurable (see also Hardin 2016a). Additionally, the methods proposed by health professionals—lose weight, change diet, take medication, exercise—were not persuasive ideas for changing health to those I knew. They felt they simply didn't have the cash to eat differently or buy medications, so what could they do? Healing chronic conditions required reflecting on interactions between health and relationships, leading Pentecostals to ask, "Who and what make it hard to change what I eat?" Salvation and healing were mirror processes—intertwined, sometimes contradictory—where the ongoingness of salvation could be measured through the ongoingness of maintaining "control" of cardiometabolic conditions. Pentecostals' healing ideologies aligned temporalities of faith and chronicity—that is "lived experiences of continuity" that "decenter the treatment of illness as a segregated, individual, and stigma-producing event" (Manderson and Smith-Morris 2010, 18). Incremental notions of faith centered on narratives of health and healing, which allowed those living with cardiometabolic disorders to decenter symptoms that came to indicate faithful flux—dizziness, hunger, numbness.

Healing, then, is not only about health, but is also a process of locating individuals within a social field, encompassing complex psychological, embodied, physical, and linguistic interactions (Csordas 2002; Mattingly and Garro 2000; Laderman and Roseman 1995; Dein 2002). Healing unfolds according to local explanatory models, which are emic understandings of the causes of disease, including ideas about what should be done to heal (Kleinman 1978, 254). Research in Spanish-speaking Latin America in particular has a rich tradition of examining explanatory models such as *susto* (fright) as a cause of diabetes.[16] Some of these models, like in Guatemala where there is a long history of state-sponsored violence, are social theories of suffering. Accordingly, *susto* caused by political violence "is not only an individual tragedy but serves as a powerful social and political record of transgressions against the indigenous population" (Green 2013, 123). *Faith and the Pursuit of Health* explores Pentecostal explanatory models to understand how ideas about what makes people sick are reflections on a changing and unequal global economy. Healing, more than explanation, is also social action, providing Pentecostals with new ways to relate to people, food, and environments. Additionally, Pentecostal healing provides two interrelated modes for accomplishing healing, that is, ritual procedures and reflection. Procedurally for Pentecostals, healing diabetes required being delivered from the spirits that caused the sickness while also reflecting on the social and individual limitations to, for example, say no to "unhealthy" but very tasty foods. This combined practice of healing rituals and reflection about the social and spiritual impetus of sickness, through practices such as prayer, is a process of locating the self in relation to powerful others—against a matrix of relationships that shape access to food, fat, and fitness. Lagi would describe this by saying, "Healing is an everyday thing. Prayer, fasting, and reading the Bible are all important. There is no formula" (see Bialecki 2007).

My adopted father's conversion narrative made this locating process clear.[17] Within hours of meeting him, Tanu explained to me that his own high blood pressure was controlled through prayer (though, months later, I would learn he also took medication). We first met at a Samoan version of Kentucky Fried Chicken—with an imitation Uncle Sam hovering above. I had expected to eat, but instead we just talked, using the table and chairs to lend structure to an encounter between strangers. Soon after, I became part of Tanu's household as his *pālagi* (white/European) daughter. He worked tirelessly with me on my language skills and offered nuanced explanations for various everyday activities, something he was accustomed to doing as he had worked as a research liaison with many New Zealand and American researchers in years past. It wasn't long before I learned that Tanu was also a performer, often leading praise and worship in the church. On my first visit to the church, Tanu surprised me by inviting me to the front of church to sing *"E Lelei le Atua"* (God is so Good) with him as a way of introducing me to the church. This succeeded in endearing me to the congregation, but not for the reasons Tanu expected. As an accomplished singer, dancer, and preacher, Tanu expected performance to be easy for me.[18] He also thought my skills in singing in Samoan would impress the congregation. Instead, my nervous, quiet "singing" inspired pity and gentle laughter, which had an equally potent (and positive) effect.

Nearly every Sunday, Tanu would talk with me after church about the sermon—explaining nuanced meaning, sometimes sharing if village events were the impetus for the sermon. We would sit in the main room watching preaching on television, or sit on the front porch drinking tea. During these chats, he would return to the story of his own conversion again and again. He "found Jesus" during a tumultuous time in his life—he was drinking, smoking, feeling sick, and "worried all the time" (see also Manderson and Kokanovic 2009). Every day, he worried that the brothers of one of the mothers of his children would find him and kill him—he had children with at least four women and had not married any of them. He felt strongly that his Catholic church permitted this kind of behavior, and ignored it, because he was a prominent youth leader—bringing "fame" to his village because of all the singing competitions he won. He would tell me that he felt "a change" when he stopped going to confession and, by extension, stopped seeking the church for forgiveness. Instead, he finally spoke directly to God saying, "I need your help." He stopped feeling so "nervous and sick all the time" when he started attending the Pentecostal church with the first woman with whom he had had children—my adopted mother. They both converted as a way of creating a "new life" together. He would say, "Thank you, God, for changing my religion."

Before Tanu converted, he felt that he was "big and fat." His wife would tease him about this, his former big belly drawing the most laughs. When he was bigger, he felt "weak, with no appetite." He was not treating his body as "the temple of God." After conversion, Tanu began to lose weight, he stopped drinking and smoking, and he began taking medication for his newly diagnosed high blood pressure. When I lived with him, he was in his seventies, and he was proud of his physical strength, which he saw as a testament to his faith—though he would attribute his strength to God, not his own ability. His spiritual practice was intimately linked to his physical fitness. Even though he had a car, once a week, Tanu would walk to the plantation (a three-mile incline) to tend to his taro plants and coconut and banana trees.

He would spend a few days at the plantation, taking "time to be close with God." Away from the business of the household and village, and without electricity, Tanu would "pray all night, sitting in the dark." The physical labor of walking and caring for the plantation was a "way to connect with God," which kept him strong while also allowing him to tend to "spiritual things." He brought this message to his family as he encouraged them to also see diet and physical fitness as a spiritual matter. One evening as we ate chicken soup with cucumbers and boiled breadfruit, Tanu scolded his young granddaughter for always picking the fatty pieces of meat from her soup, leaving the cucumbers. He said, "God is your health," and to be strong and healthy and grow, you must "eat good foods for God." Tanu also criticized his wife for "getting fat because she worries too much" about church politics and village affairs.[19]

Tanu's circuitous story speaks to the taken-for-granted ways that church was not only an institution that lent shape to everyday life, but also provided practical opportunities to come to see oneself, and others, as *persons becoming*. The ways sick persons narrated their life histories as disrupted by illness show how healing relies upon the sick person coming to terms with his or her new identity. These stories make sense of new embodied experiences of sickness. This approach is particularly evident in cases of chronic illness, where "people attempt to create continuity after . . . unexpected disruption" to their lives (Becker 1997, 4). Constructing a narrative around illness may help those living with chronic illnesses to readjust their sense of self, but uncertainty is continuous, and after treatment or diagnosis, "return to life as usual . . . is anything but 'normal'" (Moyer and Hardon 2014, 9; see also Manderson and Smith-Morris 2010; Mattingly and Garro 2000). I found sickness did not disrupt one's identity as much as it impacted one's capacity to act in the social world. Being diagnosed with diabetes, for example, meant eating differently; it required one to purchase medicine, and health practitioners encouraged people with diabetes to exercise—making people visible in the village landscape when they walked for exercise. In a place where walking, especially in the sun, was avoided, walking for exercise could be mistaken for not owning a car, or worse, not being able to afford petrol for the vehicle. So when Pentecostals came to identify as diabetic through being born again, they sidestepped the more uncomfortable social changes that often accompanied new diagnoses.

Health behaviors were difficult to implement for two reasons. First, family meals tended to be made from one pot. Therefore, changing an individual diet required change for the whole family. This led to the second change that was difficult to implement. To ask for such a change suggested that people placed their needs above that of the family. Purchasing medications was difficult for similar reasons; it required the sick person to use potentially scarce resources for individual consumption over family needs. In this way, health behaviors had social consequences that disrupted the flow of everyday life in ways that simply identifying as sick did not help to ameliorate. That is, illness transforms identity in ways that do not necessarily map onto illness identity. In this context, Pentecostal healing encouraged sick persons to highlight the development of their religious identity in day-to-day life over developing health consciousness, because changing behavior for religious reasons was more acceptable than changing behavior for health reasons.

## INTERSECTIONS, MEDICAL ANTHROPOLOGY, AND THE ANTHROPOLOGY OF CHRISTIANITY

Medical anthropologists and scholars of Christianity share an interest in analyzing healing through ritual and performance, with a historical focus on what healing "necessarily and definitively accomplishes" (Csordas 1988, 132). This was an approach I encountered as I returned from fieldwork. Scholars would often ask me if Pentecostals were "really" healthier? Were the health outcomes measurable? This approach to the accomplishments of healing rituals suggests a bias toward an empiricist approach rooted in the history of medical anthropology, beginning with Evans-Pritchard's *Witchcraft, Oracles and Magic among the Azande* (1937). From this perspective, magic and belief are a kind of dress to empirical reality, which ultimately obscures that reality. The anthropologist's task is to reveal that empirical reality, of which "the natives" are often ignorant. Anthropologists have changed course from this empiricist approach to healing to show the ways that meaning making, particularly in the form of narrative and metaphor, shapes the very reality that Evans-Pritchard sought to uncover.

This "problem of belief" is shared by medical anthropologists and scholars of Christianity.[20] A focus on belief makes it difficult to see that to be efficacious, healing does not need physical cures. Thomas Csordas's landmark work with Catholic charismatic healing in the United States makes this point clearly. By shifting analysis to embodied experience, Csordas (1988, 1993) established that healing efficacy is secured through the transformation of the dispositions of participants and their subsequent experiences of empowerment rather than of physical cure. In other words, the sickness that motivated the supplicant to seek out healing does not need to be cured for the healing to feel like it worked; through a "rhetoric of transformation," the meaning of sickness is changed (Csordas 1983). Pamela Klassen similarly argued that healing is more than a "form of bodily repair or cure" but a "rubric" used "to assess and critique" a variety of forms of healing, including Christian and biomedical (2011, 7).[21]

When Samoans interpreted chronic cardiometabolic disorders through a Pentecostal rubric, the individual body and spirit became a source of information about relationships. For example, Rita was born again when she was healed of persistent gum disease, including "pain, lots of bacteria, and little bumps," but she explained, "when I accepted the Lord, all that hate I had that was causing those problems—I gave that hate over to Him. Now I've noticed that when I feel that hate, I don't get sick anymore." She connected her feelings of "hate and anger" directed at her husband, who was drinking and gambling, with her gum disease— again linking immoral consumption with disease. When she became born again, she also underwent deliverance from the spirit of gambling and alcohol, which enabled her to "come to the Lord," thus removing the cause of her gum disease.[22] During this time, Rita saw a physician about her gums and was subsequently diagnosed with diabetes. Though Rita did not connect her oral disease with unmanaged diabetes, she didn't dispute that diabetes can cause gum disease. But her gum disease and diabetes were caused by stress from her problematic relationship with her husband. Her husband's gambling and drinking caused emotional suffering and economic precarity. Rita and her husband were often unable to make contributions to their church and family and were unable to make loan payments for their business.

A visit to the doctor and a diagnosis of diabetes and gum disease were insufficient in providing Rita with pathways to healing. Pentecostal healing showed Rita that the doctor's explanations were limited, as clinical advice disregarded the social and economic realities of her life. Rita came to bundle together her physical symptoms with the stress derived from her relationship and related economic struggle. Healing, then, was both explicitly about changing her individual body and changing her relationships, and ultimately the community, into a better Christian community—the Kingdom of God—linking salvation with mundane activities of metabolic control. Healing is more than cure; it is a critical social process. As I show in this book, Pentecostal healing brings into focus the social life of food, fat, and fitness, rendering them culturally significant symbols for expressing ambivalence about hierarchies and inequalities.

Faith, like health, is mercurial. Both are ongoing or developing, which ultimately makes flux (in body and spirit) meaningful. Health and faith are not permanently achievable states, but rather states of being that one works to achieve. Biomedicine and Christianity share an ethic of self-work and self-care; each institution encourages individuals to see themselves as projects in progress. Each, as a set of knowledges and practices, provides different tools for understanding this progress. Health metrics like weight or blood pressure provide a snapshot of complex processes occurring within the body, while Pentecostalism provides tools for seeing health as developing over time—providing a diachronic perspective. Research at the intersection of medical anthropology and the anthropology of Christianity reveals these synergies as well as the ways religious practice guides health seeking (see also Inhorn and Wentzell 2012, 19; Inhorn and Tremayne 2012).

## PLAN OF CHAPTERS

The title of this ethnography, *Faith and the Pursuit of Health: Cardiometabolic Disorders in Samoa*, refers to the two primary arguments of the book. As the first book-length ethnography of cardiometabolic disorders in Samoa—that is, an experiential analysis of the social suffering generated by and thought to cause cardiometabolic disorders, I explore the social orchestration of individual risk, showing how the individualization of risk is shared across people, community, and environment. Samoan Pentecostals highlight the social dimensions of cardiometabolic suffering by coming to see their individual symptoms as manifestations of broader social and economic change. While Samoan Pentecostals accepted the idea that food, fat, and fitness could be controlled individually, they found themselves ultimately unable to change weight, diet, or exercise—they needed to change their relationships and their community. In this book, I focus on the ways that institutions, like Christianity and biomedicine, purport individualized responsibility for risk management but, in practice, socialize risk as a community concern.

In addition, in *Faith and the Pursuit of Health*, I explore how Pentecostal healing discourses and practices provided pathways to change one's social field, and as a result, sometimes, they enabled health practices to shift as well. My goal, however, is not to suggest that Samoan Pentecostals were the only ones who recognized that social and economic suffering created conditions where cardiometabolic disorders flourished, but to suggest that Pentecostal practice provides a highly organized way to transform one's social world. Pentecostal practices globally teach people to attune their minds and bodies to become spaces where God reveals himself. In the context of rapid epidemiological change, Pentecostals used food, fat, and fitness as tools for understanding self in relation to God and human others.

In Chapter Two, I situate the reader in Samoa and describe fieldwork methods, the people and places where I spent time between clinic and church. By describing the scope of places that form the foundation for this book, my aim is to demonstrate the interstitial quality of medicine and Christianity in daily life. In Chapter Three, Discerning Ambiguous Risks, the reader is situated within some of the daily contradictions that arise around eating and feeding others when staple foods have changed, influencing the meanings of fat and fitness. I propose thinking about this process as spiritual metabolism, a framework for exploring the ways that Christianity provides pathways to create well-being, and sometimes health, by making health actions a form of religious practice. In this chapter, I also explore the globalization of cardiometabolic disorders, outlining macro political and economic changes and global trends in order to unpack how these broader dynamics are articulated in Samoa. In Chapter Four, Freedom and Health Responsibility, I focus on the everyday difficulties of refusing food or using cash resources for health reasons. Pentecostal Samoans used the language of freedom to reflect on these practical impossibilities. Freedom discourses drew attention to the social context of eating and feeding, providing some with a way to talk about the limitations of individual agency in cases when people had to accept gifts or feed others in culturally valorized ways. Pentecostals used the language of freedom to talk about the social limitations of choice and the ways that those limitations impacted health. To be free was to discursively unencumber oneself of the exigencies of social context, creating a Christian framework for both talking about the limitations of individual agency and valorizing efforts toward cultivating individual agency. Pentecostals used freedom discourses to create an epidemiological narrative that highlights the complex social, economic, and ecological interactions that create contexts where the rates of cardiometabolic disorders are so high.

In Chapter Five, I explore how fat talk about mainline pastors is a practice of embodied analytics—that is, a Pentecostal framework for understanding the signs of the body as evidence of how pastors use their wealth. What looks like fat shaming in the form of jokes about fat pastors and stories of pastoral abuse can, therefore, also be seen as embodied critique. I show how, through discussions of fat, Pentecostals scale up their etiologies from individual suffering to social suffering by throwing light on the institutional organization of wealth. In Chapter Six, Well-Being and Deferred Agency, I continue my analysis of spiritual etiologies by discussing intersections of medical events—that is, moments of diagnosis or admittance to the hospital—and conversion. When health is interpreted through the lens of Pentecostalism, new converts find tools for healing the body and changing relationships that had previously impeded them from changing health behaviors and environments. A central argument of this chapter is that conversion provides moral pathways for changing health behavior in ways that de-emphasize individual agency and foregrounded God's agency in creating health.

In Chapter Seven, Support Synergies, I show how Pentecostal theories of wellness mirror two separate veins of social science research on the impacts of social support and religious practice on health outcomes. I demonstrate that Pentecostal women generate the social support they see as lacking (and a cause of suffering) elsewhere in society. I analyze three ways in which social support and divine support were practiced together among two groups of women, a healing ministry and a women-only prayer group. First, as women taught new converts how to access God and showed women how to generate divine support, they also provided social support. Second, the social organization of women's groups fostered nonkin relationships, which deepened women's networks. Finally, the group provided a space for everyday requests for help. I argue that gendered social support mitigates stress while fostering the development of intimacy with God, both of which have been linked to wellness (see Ellison and Levin 1998).

In Chapter 8, I conclude by exploring how disease becomes the foundation for spirituality in ways that both naturalize and challenge the social and economic factors shaping the distribution of disease. Religious frameworks therefore provided a way to act that downplayed the importance of individual agency, which ultimately made some individualized action morally conceivable. This has implications for how health practitioners in Oceania frame prevention.

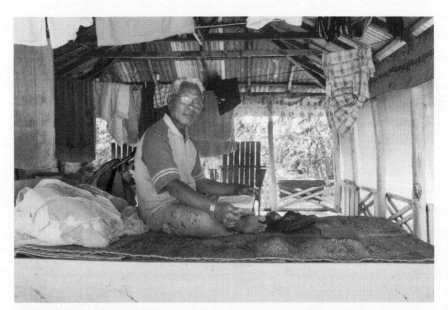

FIGURE 3 Tanu sat in his own fale on Saturdays, and after wrapping up his mosquito net and drinking morning tea, he would read his Bible. Saturday was his day to prepare for Sunday services. Most Sundays, Tanu was involved in an official manner, either shepherding the elders in their prayer before the services began, leading the praise and worship portion of the service, or offering the main sermon. The family knew not to bother him when he sat in his house, which was adjacent to the main house where everyone else slept. This space was for Tanu.

# 2 · ETHNOGRAPHY BETWEEN CHURCH AND CLINIC

Any account of health in Samoa would be incomplete without some engagement with religion, as Christianity is deeply embedded into everyday life in Samoa. Mainline churches have become thoroughly embedded within Samoan hierarchies, such that there is a Samoan-ness to the way Christianity is practiced today. Reflecting this appropriation of Christianity into a Samoan cosmology, the history of Christianity in Samoa begins with a Samoan legend—Nāfanua, the Samoan goddess of war, predicted that a new religion would come to Samoa and replace the old gods (Meleisea 1987, 57–60). Churches are intertwined with village politics as *matai* (titled political leaders, chiefs), and their families have long histories of attendance to specific churches and often serve as lay officials like deacons or elders in the church. Competition between churches reflects missionization strategies, where matai would choose a church and then entire families would convert and join the church (Meleisea 1987, 60–61).[1] Prayers open up meetings across government offices, and the Constitution of Samoa officially marks this relationship between the state and Christianity. The motto of Samoa is *Fa'avae i le Atua Samoa* (Samoa is founded on God). The national anthem also makes this clear: *Aua e te fefe; o le Atua lo ta fa'avae, o lota sa'olotoga* (Do not be afraid; God is our foundation, our freedom) (Ahdar 2013). This close relationship between politics and the church reflects how Christianity was "so completely embraced" shortly after missionaries arrived (Macpherson and Macpherson 2009, 106). In fact, the time prior to the arrival of missionaries is known as *also ole pouliuli* (days of darkness); the time after the acceptance of the gospel is referred to as *aso ole malamalama* (enlightenment) or *aso ole tala lelei* (days of the good news) (Meleisea 1987, 144).

Early church missions largely focused on education. By the 1850s, churches had established village schools, and by the 1900s, the country had achieved near universal literacy (Tuia and Schoeffel 2016). The particular missionaries who arrived in Samoa were largely working-class English and Scottish, as well as Pacific Islander, without any formal medical training (Meleisea 1987). Thus there was little explicit focus on the creation of missionary clinics, and organized care was first introduced in the 1920s by the New Zealand colonial administration. Contrasting other missionary models of medicine that linked individual sin with sickness (see Vaughan 1991), missionary medicine in Samoa focused on the agency of God to remove sickness (see Macpherson and Macpherson 1990). This mirrored how early missionaries described Samoan beliefs, with sickness and health caused by various deities (Macpherson and Macpherson 1990, 40). These early synergies are one reason that Christianity was so quickly accepted and eventually woven into Samoan cultural traditions, making any account of healing in Oceania incomplete without an understanding of religion.[2]

During my preliminary fieldwork in Hawai'i, I realized this when a pastor urged his congregants to "think outside the burger" as a way to improve "spiritual health." As a result, when conducting fourteen months of fieldwork in two villages and two churches, I came to see epidemiological change, clinical practice, and religious healing as mutually implicated. Using participant observation allowed me to contextualize what I learned in interviews—from formal life-history interviews to unstructured conversations—comparing what people said with what they did in their everyday lives. This was especially relevant around food, when people would articulate typical health promotion ideas about cutting down on foods rich with salt, fat, and sugar, and then eat and give food gifts of those same foods. Living with families, participating in church communities, and observing in healthcare spaces allowed me to see the ways prayers traveled and God emerged throughout the day. In clinics, patients prayed that God would lead doctors, while in the hospital, healers evangelized over the sick. Ethnographic methods, especially the importance of being embedded in communities over a long period of time and language learning, allowed me to work across institutional boundaries to follow my interlocutors from clinic to dinner table to church.

The longest period of fieldwork was in 2011 for fourteen months, which built upon pilot research conducted for a cumulative period of twelve months in Hawai'i (2008, 2009), American Samoa (2009), California (2010), and Samoa (2010); I conducted follow-up research in 2017. I conducted more than two hundred interviews, which can be broken down into groups: 1) patient-centered interviews in medical settings; 2) church-based network interviews; and 3) health practitioners and allied field interviews. With people from each group, I conducted repeat interviews. Some interviews, particularly those with health practitioners who were also in my church network, are included in both groups; in these cases, interview guides were combined.

Patient-centered interviews in medical settings include semistructured interviews at a diabetes clinic, dialysis center, and district hospitals; the data set includes fifty-nine interviews conducted predominantly in Samoan with the help of a research assistant. These lasted anywhere from twenty minutes to one hour. I developed the interview guide with my research assistant and tested it several times before using it in the clinics. Church-based network interviews were semistructured and open ended. These interviews lasted anywhere from thirty minutes to three hours. This group includes eighty-six interviews. I recruited individuals for these interviews primarily via word of mouth. The interviewee determined the interview location—sometimes over coffee, sitting on the seawall, or in church buildings.

I conducted ninety-nine semistructured interviews with health practitioners and those working in allied fields in aid or with NGOs. I worked with diverse health professionals for the entire fieldwork period. I interviewed at the United Nations and World Health Organization offices, had coffee with public health volunteers from Australia, and regularly used the library at the Ministry of Health (MOH). I interviewed physicians, nurses, policy authorities, and aid workers. The initial recruitment was a purposive sampling method. I first developed a list of organizations and institutions to target and then employed the snowball method to recruit the remaining interviewees. Interviews were conducted in English or Samoan, depending on the interviewee preference. I audio and video recorded in various settings in order to complement narrative-based data in interviews. I audio recorded at the diabetes clinic, churches, and Bible study and prayer meetings. This data also documents the same individuals in diverse settings, from ritual events, like baptisms, to casual prayers that followed. I collected the newspaper during long-term fieldwork and read the previous two year's back issues. I also kept a food log of household meals and the foods entering and exiting my households.

During preliminary fieldwork, my interview guides were predominantly focused on cardiometabolic disorder knowledge; I wanted to know what people knew about the symptoms and causes of diabetes. I found these interviews were often very flat; in other words, participants easily recited the causes of diabetes as related to diet and exercise. When I changed my interview guide to include questions about spirituality, or the connections between spiritual health and physical health, the interviews became more candid. I started to ask people about their churches, and if they were born again, and why and when they had changed their church. These questions extended interviews from quick fifteen-minute interactions to hour or longer affairs. Interview participants often noted that they enjoyed discussing their health and causes of stress in their everyday lives. As a result of this preliminary research, long-term fieldwork was designed to include equal time in church, households, and clinics—places I describe below.

## TWO CHURCHES, TWO HOUSEHOLDS

The Assemblies of God (AOG) church was peachy brown; it was faded and the concrete chipped. Painted prominently on the front of the church was an image of angels with a banner reading, "Where the Christians Meet." Later, I would learn that the balcony would shake from the bass of the praise and worship team. While conventional churches—what were locally referred to as mainline churches, such as Congregational, Methodist, and Catholic churches—still maintain the majority of church congregations, *lotu fou* (new churches) have been growing in terms of individual identification and the number of churches established (see Ernst 2012; Pagaialii 2006).[3] However, these groups have faced difficulties in establishing churches because village councils control village lands, and therefore they control what can be built on them. Church divisions tend to follow social divisions derived from matai because, through the village council, they control the number and types of churches permitted to practice within their villages (Meleisea 1987; Va'ai 2012). This is significant because, historically, matai have been associated with the mainstream churches. Until recently, families who chose to leave mainline churches faced discrimination and in some cases even banishment from villages. Yet despite the initial difficulties in establishing new churches, there has been a slow exodus from mainline churches to Pentecostal churches for two reasons: changed worship styles and giving practices (Thornton, Kerslake, and Binns 2010).

The AOG church was technically in a neighboring village to my adopted family's five-room house, which sat shaded by a seemingly ancient mango tree. When I first stayed with my adopted family during pilot research in 2010, the house did not have any windows, it was a hybrid *fale Samoa* (a Samoan house without walls) in the front—a raised concrete platform with an arched roof supported by poles made of small painted tree trunks—and in the back, there were three small bedrooms. When I returned a year later for long-term fieldwork, the house had been transformed into a *fale pālagi* (a European house, with walls). The poles had been replaced with louver windows and concrete walls painted bright yellow and turquoise, which reflected the fact that the daughter had graduated from university and had started working, so she could contribute to the renovations. The house was on the main road that snaked the coast from the capital, Apia, to the airport to the wharf. Behind the house was a small plantation—with a few coconut, papaya, and breadfruit trees in addition to leafy greens, cucumbers, and aromatic leaf trees used for tea. The family also kept a small gated area with a few pigs—let to grow fat in case an especially important event arose. At dusk, right before the *sā* (the evening prayer time), the pigs were permitted to wander as young men played rugby or girls played volleyball. Each evening in households across Samoa, families gather to say evening prayers. The ringing of a village bell, the hitting of a metal object, or the blowing of a large empty shell by the local pastor are all possible cues to signal the start of the evening period called *sa* (meaning both "sacred" and "forbidden"). At this time, children and adults who were still on the road would rush home or, if that were not possible, stop by the house of the closest friends or relatives to turn their attention to the *lotu* (the evening prayer). In some villages, traffic on the road is stopped by the *'aumaga* (village organization of untitled men), and those found outside during sā can be fined.

In the mornings before the sun rose, I could hear waves crashing the seawall and the sounds of buses loudly breaking as they stopped for people waving them down. Like others in my household, I commuted to Apia in the mornings on

crowded buses with schoolteachers, civil servants, workers employed in the former auto parts manufacturing factory, and those shopping. Buses would fill up
with plastic bags from the supermarkets in town or palm baskets filled with
vegetables, starches, or coconuts bought from roadside agricultural stalls run by
families. My own AOG household, like all the families who were part of the congregation, maintained family plantations. When I first started learning about
Samoa, I envisioned plantations as large areas of land, densely planted in organized rows. Family plantations, however, are more like large gardens. Families
sometimes maintained two different kinds of gardens, a starch-based plantation
of banana trees, taro plants, and breadfruit trees, and a garden of fruit trees like
papaya, coconut, and mango and vegetables like cucumber, tomato, and cabbage.
Sometimes households would have a garden at their house while also maintaining
family lands elsewhere with more of the same foods.

Households on the northwest side where I lived were crowded with family
members from distance villages as they sought to work or go to school in Apia,
which made villages on this side of the island larger than more rural villages. One
consequence of this increasing density is there is less space near the house to grow
a garden, requiring families to cultivate plantations inland, away from the village.
This is challenging due to transport and time constraints, and the ever present fear
of people stealing food from the plantation. As you drive the main road of Upolu,
the most noticeable structures you encounter are churches and *fale talimalo*—
large houses for each of the matai in the village, which are left open and ready for
occupancy by visitors, usually used when hosting large family events. These structures are abundant, and even when churches are out of sight, signs on the main
road mark congregations that have established churches inland. The landscape of
concrete block and open-air wooden fale were dwarfed by multistory, often crisply
painted church edifices, which speak to the rhythm of the week that was set by
the church: Sunday school meetings, church elders meetings, special prayer calls,
Wednesday evening services, four-o'clock-in-the-morning private prayer calls, and
two Sunday services. These services were in addition to any special arrangements
required for holidays like Mother's Day or Christmas when extensive perfor-
mances were often organized.

Established in the 1980s, the AOG church was one of fourteen churches located
in a village of roughly 3,700 people (Village Population 2016). This was the first
AOG church in the village, and it attracted families from neighboring villages without Pentecostal churches in their own villages. The AOG services were lively—
the praise and worship team played popular Samoan and English Pentecostal
songs, the congregants danced enthusiastically, and, during the sermon, they
called out *sa'o lelei* (that's true), hallelujah, and *amene* when they agreed. The worship at this AOG church was marked by its excitement, rather than by charismatic manifestations of the Holy Spirit. Music, dancing, and clapping created a
celebratory atmosphere. A few congregants were known to be "stronger believers,"

and while others prayed quietly, with their eyes closed, heads down, or swayed to beats of the praise and worship team, they occasionally collapsed or burst into glossolalia. These were rare occasions, not totally welcome but not totally unexpected. Many, most notably the pastor, maintained that charismatic practices had been routinized, which was seen as a kind of accomplishment. The "fire" of the Holy Spirit was strongest, the logic went, when the missionaries first arrived, and then again in the 1970s and 1980s when Pentecostal churches started to grow in Samoa. Today, however, these AOG congregants were *masani* (accustomed) to the Holy Spirit and were "mature" Christians.

In contrast to the AOG church, the church I call Glory House was one of the most charismatic churches in Samoa; the church website reports having eight thousand members, although its pastors suggested that the active membership was closer to two thousand members. The church had offices in Apia, in one of the few remaining wood buildings adjacent to the missionary school also established by the church. The congregation met in the national gymnasium, which was transformed each week into a worship space, as band equipment, projectors for song lyrics, flowers, and cell groups brought in bolts of fabric for decoration.[4] These cell groups met locally each week, in villages where there were enough congregation members to start their own group. These groups typically met in a family home, or, in other cases, in the back rooms of family-owned stores. In addition to cell group meetings, congregants were expected to do periodic fundraising, "sausage sizzles," for example, or participate in evangelism trips to villages without cell groups, and attend regular events like the annual healing services.

The church was largely organized around a charismatic pastor who was raised a Methodist and converted. He started a tent revival in Apia in the 1990s, which figured heavily in the conversion narratives of Samoans of a certain age from various church denominations. Church members largely came from the greater Apia area, although church buses brought families from more distant villages as well. There were nine satellite churches on the two islands (Upolu and Savai'i), each with pastors. These satellite churches joined the main congregation periodically. A few congregations were close enough to Apia to join the "mother church" regularly for evening services. This church attracted a diverse membership, ranging from displaced individuals—those banished from their villages for wanting to worship in a Pentecostal church—to urban elites.

Each of these churches attracted an economically diverse congregation—ranging from those who worked their plantations and sold their agricultural goods to teachers and government workers. The households I lived in also ranged from modest to relatively affluent. The AOG household included my adopted mother and father, both of whom were titled village leaders, their married daughter, her husband and small children, their unmarried son (a young man in his twenties), and their eight-year-old granddaughter (the daughter of their son who lived in New Zealand). They had three additional sons who lived in New Zealand and one daughter who was a *faletua* (a pastor's wife) on the more rural island of Savai'i.[5] There were many cash flows into the household with two matai, two working household members (the daughter was a school teacher; her husband worked in a government office), remittances from New Zealand, and regular gifts from the faletua. However, it was not uncommon for the electricity to go out or for the pickup truck to be out of commission because there was no money for petrol. Even with remittances and salaries, cash demands far exceeded collective earnings.

In the town area, tucked behind the main road, a Catholic secondary school, and village plantations, was the home of my second host family. My first introduction to the household quickly immersed me into the charisma of daily life with Lagi. She was late picking me up on the day I moved in because she had organized a "deliverance" for her friend the night before, which kept her awake until the early morning. Lagi lived with her husband and three small children in a newly built home on freehold land.[6] They were successful in their jobs, with desirable positions in prominent businesses, consistent with their overseas education. They spoke predominantly English at home, except when speaking to their housekeeper, and they attended the English-speaking congregation of Glory House. All of these factors were typical of an emerging urban elite in Samoa.

Lagi's mother and brother lived on an adjacent plot. Each of Lagi's siblings owned a plot, creating something akin to village life, but Lagi and her mother were the only ones to have built homes. Lagi's mother and brother attended their former village-based Catholic church—driving over an hour each Sunday to attend church. This denominational diversity was a source of almost daily tension and negotiation. While Lagi's mother was embarrassed that her daughter had left the family church, Lagi was deeply concerned that her mother had not been born again. Lagi organized events at her house that were often geared toward generating ambient Christianity through a charismatic soundscape as a way to influence her mother (Engelke 2013; Hirschkind 2006; Feld 1982), saying things like, "If she hears us, maybe the Holy Spirit will move her."

The population in Samoa is increasingly urban, with the villages surrounding the town area growing as quickly as the Apia population. Working with churches in the periphery of town, as well as in town, provided me with access to a range of people from those who were subsistence farmers and experiencing cash poverty, unable to pay for life's necessities like school fees or electricity, to professionals working in the formal economy with no gardens, who felt burdened by having to purchase all of their foods in addition to other required expenses. I also participated and observed daily conversations and practices of reciprocity as I watched fundraising raffle sales, cases of food come and go, and late evening visits by family members soliciting resources. Lagi's mother would sometimes knock on our door in the very early morning to ask for money for a fa'alavelave or to remind Lagi that a relative would be visiting, which meant she needed to be sent back to her village with something like food or money. In my AOG household, matai would often arrive after the evening meal, which would require the quick manifestation of food. When a guest arrived, my adopted niece would run to the village store to buy a loaf of bread and butter. The older siblings would quickly cut the bread, make a cup of milky sugary tea, find a tray, move a table to the visitor, and then, gracefully, serve this tray to the visitor. I was consistently amazed at how quickly—even when there was no food in the house because there was no cash—a tray, table, food, and drink could be mustered to appropriately accept a request for contributions to family projects.

## HOSPITALS, CLINICS, AND PUBLIC HEALTH OFFICES

Each day as my family members went to work, I also left the house to work in clinics, the national hospital, or public health offices. Much of my time was spent in the MOH offices, located across the road from the main hospital. Newly painted and recently built with the help of Chinese aid, the building shimmered white. The air-conditioned offices housed various divisions responsible for strategic health planning, disease surveillance, and health promotion. Whether interviewing those working on noncommunicable diseases or nutrition, or reading policy documents in the library, the MOH offices provided a window into how global health paradigms were localized in Samoa (see also Keshavjee 2014; Farmer, Kim, Kleiman, and Basilico 2013; Biehl and Petryna 2013). The policy division of healthcare was distinct from providers and clinical services, which were offered across the road at one main location, the Tupua Tamasese Mea'ole Hospital.[7] There were also smaller district clinics staffed by local nurses, with visiting physicians in clinic only a few days a week.

The government is currently focused on improving primary care—that is district hospitals—because of long waits at the capital hospital in addition to the perceived effect that travel to the main hospital has on delaying presentation of sicknesses of all kinds (Likou 2015). The government aims to enhance the district hospitals, which means increasing staff and the regular availability of supplies—most pharmacies were stocked each day by delivery from the capital, which meant there were often shortages of pharmaceuticals and other basic supplies. In 2016, the government opened its first primary healthcare center in the capital, in what were the original buildings of the main hospital built in the 1970s.[8] The national emphasis on primary care is largely a function of attempting to implement a prevention model of noncommunicable disease management. The ministry recently defined its guiding principles as "Health Promotion" and "Primary Health Care," showing that health education is seen as a complement to strengthening primary care (Ministry of Health 2012). This effort is guided by policy that seeks to integrate private, public, global, and NGO health services to address gaps in healthcare staffing, infrastructure, and supplies (Ministry of Health 2010).

This focus on primary healthcare is not new to Samoa; in fact, the initial healthcare provisioning organized by the New Zealand colonial administration was organized around a model of community-based primary care. The administration organized rural women into associations called *komiti tumama* as the "backbone of public programs," playing a critical role in preventive medicine at the village level (Schoeffel 1984, 209). The colonial administration was motivated by two factors: domestic policy was focused on developing primary care and responding to the influenza epidemic, which in 1918 killed somewhere between 20 percent and 22 percent of the population in Samoa (Boyd 1980; Tomkins 1992). Women's organizations, although an invention of colonial administration, are still today viewed as essential cultural institutions (see also Fairbairn-Dunlop 1998). The initial organizations were highly effective because they were largely operated autonomously from colonial administrators and raised the status of the married women who participated in them, thereby increasing the women's commitment to such services. The associations decreased in effectiveness in the early 1980s as the government shifted focus from autonomous village organizations to centralization and professionalization of national health services. This shift, combined with other rapid social and economic changes, including the stagnation of rural village economies, decreased the status of these women's associations. With professionalization and centralization came a sense among women's committees that responsibility for health and well-being lay with the government, not the village.

Another important detractor from the role of women's organizations in preventive medicine is what Penelope Schoeffel (1984) calls the "ritualization" of certain key preventive tasks, such as village sanitation inspections. This remains a central dilemma in health promotion design today, finding strategies that incorporate village leaders into service delivery in ways that meet the needs of the program as well as the villages. Sanitation inspections provide a good example of the differing interests of the state and villages in conceptions of health. While sanitary inspections were designed to ensure the appropriate disposal of waste, a successful inspection became a source of village pride and competition over the aesthetics of villages. The associations were known to focus on the visible dimensions of sanitation while neglecting nonappearance-based issues. For example, refuse was dumped in one village behind outhouses and out of view, or thrown into the lagoon, or piles of coconut shells breeding mosquitos in nonpublic spaces were not considered problematic. The appearance of the village was considered the significant indicator of wellness because it reflected the ability of the community to work together.

One consequence of centralization has been a general decline in the status of district hospitals as primary care providers. People often told me they avoided the clinics and preferred the main hospital because there they were guaranteed to see a physician. However, getting to the hospital, located in Apia, could require sometimes lengthy travel. While preferable to local clinics, the hospital was still a place that, as Malae, a physician who taught at the medical school, described it, was "pretty grim." This was especially true of the "acute ward" where he told me to expect to see people who had "never managed" their cardiometabolic disorders— where "people go to die." In addition, most healthcare providers I talked with thought that Samoans only came to the hospital when the symptoms or health problem had seriously progressed. Patients and providers reported that people would turn to traditional medicine first, seeking out a *taulasea* (traditional healer) when they felt dizzy or had a wound that wouldn't heal (see Macpherson 1985; Macpherson and Macpherson 1990; Suaalii-Sauni et al. 2014). By the time people came to the hospital, prevention of further complications or cure were often no longer possible.

Resembling a tropical relic, the hospital was a deteriorating, white-washed concrete building with louver windows. The entry to the acute ward had a central corridor that divided the space into two sides. Each side, without partitions or walls, had multiple beds, perhaps three or four cramped next to each other. The walls were covered with hanging tubes disconnected from absent medical technology and empty shelves. Individuals were required to bring their own attendant, usually an unemployed family member, to provide basic services like bathing, feeding, cleaning sheets, and assistance with toileting. Thus, next to each bed was at least one family member, if not more, who slept on the floor. If the family were lucky, they were located next to the balcony where caretakers could sleep outside on mats. *Lāvalava* draped benches and tables crowded between beds; food covered with netting was stacked next to cellphones and Bibles. Without fans, there was a stench, and during the rainy season, it was uncomfortably hot. Stories abounded of death at the hospital and the evil spirits that eagerly watched operations in the surgical theater.

The hospital stood in notable contrast to the diabetes clinic, which was full of flowers, music, and the charismatic warmth of the head nurse. As a result, and especially given the reputation of the hospital, the clinic was an inviting medical facility. The diabetes clinic was the only clinic providing diabetes-focused primary care and was managed by a trailblazing nurse practitioner, Mele. Patients were referred to the clinic from the hospital when their blood sugar tested high. Mele would hold orientation sessions with new patients, spending up to an hour with them. She would then schedule monthly, or sometimes weekly, appointments depending on their "control."[9]

Mele carefully orchestrated the waiting area to create a relaxing space, which she hoped would encourage patients to return. Mele also wanted to ensure the patients had "peace of mind" so their suka and toto had time to return to normal levels after the morning stress of travel to the clinic. To this end, the only nonmedical member of the staff played a keyboard (borrowed from Mele), while patients waited to see the doctors; patients would often sing, and sometimes even dance, while they waited. Another way Mele tried to create a peaceful environment was by opening the clinic with a prayer. Each morning, Mele would select the eldest man, or eldest woman if there was no man, to lead the group in a prayer

(Hardin 2016b). The prayers varied in length from a few minutes to over ten minutes. The prayers often reminded the crowded waiting area of patients that the medicines the doctors and nurses provided were only effective because of God. "Our lives are in your hands. You are the living God. God, we call on you to shine your love upon us who are gathered here in this house. Our fathers and our mothers, we carry them to you through the hands of doctors and nurses who are helping them get better. Bless all of them. We remember the ministry that your healing *mana* (sacred power) comes through the medicine they have prepared."

After the prayer, the group would sing one of a few common hymns, then Mele would close the prayer by saying, "To God be the glory, forever and ever, amen," while she pumped her fist in the air—indexing her Pentecostal identity. After prayers, Mele offered education sessions while patients waited to see the doctor, explaining the physiological dimensions of diabetes or the importance of regularly taking medication.

## A NOTE ON POSITIONALITY

I study fat in Samoa: how people describe it, how health practitioners try to eliminate it, and how best to eat it, or avoid it.[10] I am not, however, by Samoan standards, fat. How then, as a "thin" woman, could I learn about fat without influencing how my interlocutors responded to my questions about fat, and food and fitness? Similarly, how did my status as "raised Catholic" (i.e., not born again) influence the way Pentecostals talked to me about faith? In both instances, instead of limitations, these aspects of my identity opened up the possibilities for learning about my interlocutors' perspectives.

In the first instance, my body (and my fat) was a method for learning. My changing weight and tastes became a source of learning both about my Samoan interlocutors and about my American friends, family, and colleagues. When I began fieldwork, I had room to grow (by Samoan standards), and, with a desire to be liked, I ate my way through fieldwork, gaining weight during each preliminary fieldwork trip. I was encouraged and complimented for such changes by my Samoan interlocutors—a source of pleasurable commentary. However, later in fieldwork, I began losing weight, which made for uncomfortable family meals when my adopted family grew concerned for my well-being, often nudging food to me during meals or sympathetically saying *kalo fai* (what a pity) when they saw me in my once formfitting puletasi. In contrast, my friends and family in the United States met me at airports, dinner parties, and conferences with zeal: "You look fantastic!" or "How did you lose weight?"

My growing interest in eating fatty foods like tinned corned beef with white rice and the slices of fat that accompanied pig roasts generated interest from my interlocutors, colleagues, and family alike. During one Sunday lunch where I enthusiastically filled my plate, the pastor noticed and announced to the group that I was clearly a "white girl with a brown heart." In another instance, the sight of me snacking on boiled bananas while driving to the beach for a BBQ elicited such joyful attention that my friend pointed at me, snapped a photo, and alerted her father, who was driving, saying, "Look, she likes bananas!" In contrast, when talking with friends and family about fieldwork, they frequently asked about why the "obesity epidemic" was happening in the islands. When I explained the effects of shifting global food trade and labor patterns, conversations often turned to discussions about fast food and the presumed cultural imperialism that was thought to accompany the establishment of restaurants like McDonalds. "How did you eat?" people asked, or "Did you *really* like the food?"

I tried to quell concerns by talking about the tasty qualities of foods that typically triggered a great deal of disgusted interest—foods like corned beef seemed to occupy the most attention. These reactions—what I have come to see as delighted disgust—crystalize the ideas that Mary Douglas explored nearly forty years ago: "Disgust and fear are taught, they are put into the mind by culture" (1975, ix). From these conversations, I came to see disgust about food as a mask for disgust about fat. Food talk, in this context, was acceptable fat talk. Sometimes, fat talk was more direct. When I was meeting with an acupuncturist via Skype, she asked about my weight, saying, "You look pretty puffy and heavy." Knowing that I did research in Samoa, she sympathetically asked, "Did you gain weight in Samoa?" I asked that we not talk about weight, explaining some ideas from the Health at Every Size movement. Backtracking a bit, she said she "admired" my "confidence in my body" but was "deeply concerned because even though most women in Samoa are obese, it doesn't mean they are healthy. They are sick. They just don't know it." I was quite disturbed by this interaction; needless to say, this was my last encounter with her. This kind of response was common, suggesting the entrenched notion that fat is dangerous and sickness inevitable (Rothblum and Solovay 2009; McCullough and Hardin 2013).

My religious identity also shaped both my interactions in Samoa and how my research was understood in the United States. My "unsaved" status made me a potential convert to some—an attractive interlocutor, one who could be taught. My status as "raised Catholic" was enough to make me trustworthy. While religious affiliation was less of a concern among my colleagues, researchers tended to be interested in the empirical dimensions of my research. Does fasting *really* help people lose weight? Once Samoans convert, do they have better control of their diabetes? This line of questioning often implicitly suggested that the only value of religious participation was if it resulted in physical results; otherwise these converts had been duped.

In this way, both my body and my religious identity became a source of data. Following Ira Bashkow, who used his whiteness as "a powerful methodology" to understand perceptions of race in Papua New Guinea, I attempted to "discover how my own world was perceived by my .. research subjects" by virtue of our perceived differences (2006, 15). I sketch out these contrasts to empirically and ethnographically ground the ways that my identity shaped the research process, but also to reflect on how cultural prototypes of fatness, Pacific Islanders, and Pentecostalism shaped my analysis. Susan Harding (1991), one of the first anthropologists to study Pentecostalism in the United States, pointed to this when she argued that fundamental Christians tend to be represented as oppositional to the modern subject. She writes, "From the modern point of view, the word 'fundamentalist' conjures up a jumbled and troubling universe of connotations, clichés, images, feelings, poses, and plots: militant, strident, dogmatic, ignorant, duped, backward, rural, southern, uneducated, antiscientific, anti-intellectual, irrational, absolutist, authoritarian, reactionary, bigoted, racist, sexist, anticommunist, war mongers" (Harding 1991, 373). The word "obese" conjures a similarly "troubling universe" of meaning: lazy, immoral, stupid, poor, unhealthy, ignorant, lacking self-control, diseased, and ugly (Greenhalgh 2012; Brewis et al. 2011; McCullough 2013). In the United States, the "obesity epidemic" suggests national decline, "eroding the nation's health, emptying its coffers, and threatening its security by depriving it of fit military recruits" (Greenhalgh 2012, 5). The fat subject thus counters a model of responsible citizenship, and in this light, the Fat Other is also a kind of "repugnant Other" (Harding 1991). The polarities generated in casual conversations about my research helped to form divisions between "us" and "them," and by extension fat and fundamental, secular and fit. My research, by dint of topic, inadvertently reproduces these global discourses about the dangers of fat and is one example of how fat subjectification spreads globally (Greenhalgh 2012). Hence, this is as much a story about how Pentecostal Christians interpret fat and cardiometabolic disorders as it is a story about the contemporary context of fat shame and loathing that animates the vast background of media, research, and politics (see also West 2005).

The history of my research in Samoa also shaped this project in multiple ways. For many months, I faced roadblocks when approaching various health institutions. In daily interactions when health officials, public health staff, or physicians did not show up to a scheduled appointment or return my calls, I came to see how "research," especially health research, was a word with a loaded history in Samoa. Linda Tuhiwai Smith (1999, 1) captures this clearly when she writes, "The term 'research' is inextricably linked to European imperialism and colonialism. The word itself, 'research,' is probably one of the dirtiest words in the indigenous world's vocabulary. When mentioned in many indigenous contexts, it stirs up silence, it conjures up bad memories, it raises a smile that is knowing and distrustful."[11]

Smith's observation draws attention to the weight of research—both the word "research" and project of research—especially for a non-Samoan nonislander in Samoa. On the one hand, research was welcomed by and readily understandable to almost all the Samoans I encountered. Research on *fa'asāmoa* (the Samoan way, Samoan culture), for example, was considered appropriate. It generated interest, support, and the resources of time. Tanu, my adoptive father, for instance, would introduce me to elders in the village when I expressed interest in fa'asāmoa, and sat with me for hours recounting Samoan oral traditions. From his perspective, research was an activity focused on documenting worlds that were alternative to those of the West, and ultimately valorized difference. On the other hand, research into potentially negative aspects of everyday life—sexuality, disease, conflict, violence—was often regarded with suspicion. My research was deemed to be somewhere between appropriate and undesirable: interest in Christianity was a desirable project, one that would bring attention to Samoa as a Christian nation, while research on cardiometabolic disorders was treated with greater reservation. This in part reflects the history of anthropology in Samoa.

I learned early in my fieldwork not to identify as an anthropologist because anthropology seemed inevitably to trigger discussions of Margaret Mead. When my interlocutors would sometimes joke about me being the "next Margaret Mead," it was not a compliment. While Mead is famed in the United States as the first public anthropologist, in Samoa, her legacy is tainted by the content of her findings. Never was this clearer than when I read *Coming of Age in Samoa* (Mead 1928a) with my anthropology students at the National University of Samoa. Initially, they were suspicious of Mead although they did not know exactly why; like others I met, the students had heard various things about her. Some were intimately familiar with the controversy surrounding Derek Freeman's claim that Mead had been "hoaxed," while others felt sympathy for Mead who had fallen for the hijinks of young girls (Freeman 1983, 1991, 1999; Caton 1990).[12] Still others recounted rumors that Mead was probably mentally ill—a few mentioned that they had heard she walked around New York City with a cape and staff as evidence of this. Others had simply heard of anthropology because of Mead. Some knew there was a controversial history, but they did not know what about; some felt that Mead had maliciously lied to make herself famous.

When my students read her book, they felt that she had described life in Samoa in ways that seemed true—until they reached the chapters about sexuality. Then they became uncomfortable. Mead's claims that Samoa was a place of youthful sexual exploration made many question the validity of anthropological methods where people could lie and anthropologists could exaggerate. Paul Shankman writes, "For some Samoans, the problem with Mead was not only *what* she wrote about their private lives but *that* she wrote about them without their knowledge or approval" (2009, 136). The wide reach of *Coming of Age* made "Samoans acutely aware of the risks of sharing their traditions with outsiders" (italics original, Shankman 2009, 142). Another concern was that *Coming of Age in Samoa* was written for lay American audiences, not Samoans. The basic questions of the book are geared toward cross-cultural comparison—that adolescent development need not be as stressful as it is (or was) in the United States. The rhetorical strategy of this book—to understand "the West" by coming to Samoa—is articulated when Mead

(1928b, 6–7) writes, "I have tried to answer the question which sent me to Samoa: Are the disturbances which vex our adolescents due to the nature of adolescence itself or to the civilization? Under different conditions does adolescence present a different picture?" Answering American questions with stories collected about life in Samoa contributed to the sense that I encountered in my own research, that researchers "take" from Samoa but do not often give back.

Overall, the history of research in Samoa is one where the directionality of data—meaning information about Samoans, their culture and bodies—has been used to produce knowledge that sometimes stigmatizes Samoans themselves. This reflects the colonial legacy embedded in research practices that demonstrate the binary between researcher and researched, "between knowing inquirer and who or what are considered to be the resources or grounds for knowledge production" (TallBear 2014, 1). This is something scholars working to forge an indigenous anthropology in Oceania aim to address when they write about decolonizing research (Tengan, Ka'ili, and Fonoti 2010; Anae 2010; Smith 1999; see also West 2016). Some scholars argue that creating scholarship that addresses "the compelling questions" of particular communities while initiating "discussions about how to address local challenges" is one step toward decolonizing research (Barker and Fonoti 2010, 308). In an effort to think with indigenous scholars and their allies, I purposely did not approach this topic in terms of health knowledge, but instead I followed my interlocutors' lead to learn how they found meaningful ways to talk about and act upon cardiometabolic disorders. I explore how Pentecostals are themselves analysts of inequalities. It is not that Pentecostals are committed to social justice (although some are), but that their healing efforts brought into focus how social and economic suffering generated sickness.

I aim to think anthropologically with a "commitment to the well-being of those being researched" by looking to how the Pentecostals I knew strove to create well-being (Hereniko 2000, 88). I will never "truly know what it is like to be Samoan," as Albert Wendt has written (quoted in Shankman 2009, 137). He cautions that outsiders "must not pretend they can write from inside us'" (Wendt 1987, 89; quoted in Hereniko 2000, 89). Instead, my research follows the expertise of people I met, from Bible study to emergency prayer calls and hospitals through food markets, pharmacies, clinics, and healing services.

Moving between clinical and religious spaces revealed the synergies in domains that are sometimes contrasted as distinct. The Western dichotomy separating belief from reason, body from mind, faith from knowledge, material from immaterial, God from medicine, creates boundaries regularly troubled by anthropologists (see Corwin and Hardin forthcoming; Finkler 1984, 1994; Whitmarsh and Roberts 2016). As an ethnographer, I sought out spaces where these contrasts were clearly dissolved. In this book, I show the shared logics in biomedicine and Christianity, even while exploring how Pentecostal approaches to health and healing point to the limitations of biomedicine.

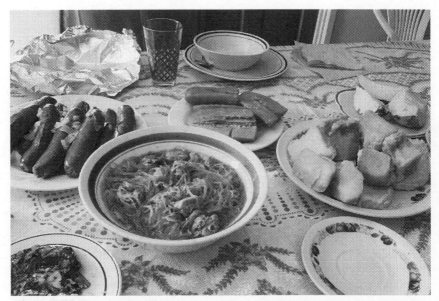

FIGURE 4 My stomach grumbled during services every Sunday. When the services were finished, the family eagerly jumped in the truck to return home, knowing there was food waiting for us. While most of the family went to church, the youngest son stayed back. He finished the umu (earth oven), which had been prepared by the men at 3 AM. The men would heat the rocks, drink tea, and wait for the banana, taro, and breadfruit to cook. Sometimes they would fill halved coconuts with coconut cream and tinned fish to cook in the oven as well, making a sweet and salty custardy sauce. These essential Sunday items paired best with lu'au, or what is called palusami when you serve it to a matai—baby taro leaves smothered in coconut cream, also slow cooked in the umu. Meat was also necessary: fish could be cooked in the umu, or chicken enveloped in sugar and soy sauce and baked in the oven, usually cooked by the women in the house before they left for church. Locally made sausages might be fried with onions, though when a container with onions was lost at sea and there were no onions on the island for a month, we skipped the sausages.

# 3 · DISCERNING AMBIGUOUS RISKS

At morning tea at the diabetes clinic, I sat behind a screen draped in fabric with brightly colored hibiscus flowers in the two-room clinic with John, a Samoan physician, while he explained the major cause of cardiometabolic disorders in Samoa. These disorders were a problem of "access to a lifestyle where you cannot pick your own food." His explanation was surprising to me, given that most families in Samoa had access to land, and therefore, food they could grow themselves. When I asked about this, he shifted the topic, saying, "My own battle is with food, because we are family oriented and I find that I am healthiest when I am overseas working." He found himself "pining for healthy foods" at home when eating with his family because he felt these dinners lacked fruits and vegetables— something he associated with health, in contrast with the meat- and starch-based dinners his family ate. He felt he was "healthier" when he was traveling because he *chose* his own foods.

Samoan physicians and nurses frequently discussed everyday eating habits as contrary to good health practices such as controlling food intake. Adapting to family dinners, as John did, was bad for health even if it was good for family relationships. Raising a slightly different point, one physician, trying to explain why his patients didn't change their diets, said: "What I am saying is, they eat those fatty foods every day. They know they should be eating differently, but it's the fa'asamoa. We just don't have a culture of vegetable eating. I try to counsel on the importance of prioritizing health, but you know a lot of the time, they prioritize other things. If there's little money, it will be for the church instead of, you know, going to the hospital or buying vegetables. Even though there are changes, in health and whatnot, they keep their values."

Both of these physicians pointed to how social expectations shaped eating, leading individuals to choose what was best for the family over what was best for individual health—what they would refer to as fa'asamoa. In this way, individual health and family well-being were positioned as opposites. In the context of Oceania, well-being has been long established as related to kin relations (Macpherson and Macpherson 1990; Parsons 1985; Manuela and Sibley 2015; McLennan 2015; Moore, Leslie, and Lavis 2005; McMullin 2010). Clinical practice was not equipped to address the social dimensions of eating, physical activity, and weight loss that were often considered "barriers" to behavior change. For example, John was hoping to start a program called "KYN," an acronym for "Know Your Numbers." He wanted all of his patients to have a "report card" as part of their medical records, recording important cardiometabolic metrics like blood pressure and weight. He felt this knowledge would change behavior precisely because these numbers de-emphasized the social dimensions of eating and highlighted how individuals might control their diet to impact their health. These kinds of explanations about the rise in cardiometabolic disorders focused on the problem of individuals becoming responsible for their own health, a choice that medical practitioners felt should be prioritized over family well-being.

Pentecostals also recognized an individualized model of health responsibility, which I realized early on while at a Glory House service. We always sat high in the stadium seats to the side of the collapsible stage, which on this evening was flanked with red ginger floral arrangements and draped in sequined maroon fabric. The praise and worship team wore matching maroon floral clothing and as the pastor walked on stage, with his matching shirt and white shell *lei*, he touched the bellies of the elders who stood nearby—hands raised, singing with the praise of worship team. Lagi brought me to church this particular midweek evening to participate in a special series focused on healing. She had participated the previous year and had "advanced spiritually" during the event—she was "slain" for the first time, meaning that, as a pastor touched her, she fell to the ground. That night the pastor preached about "curses" as a source of sickness because, he felt, "Samoa is a country that is really good at cursing. The people enjoy cursing other people, especially the relationship between parents and children, between the church and the pastor." The pastor claimed he could "help" Samoa by instructing the attendees on deliverance methods. The pastor said flatly, "Jesus came to deliver you" and the Bible instructs on how: "This is not the teachings of our church, or my own. It's the teachings of the Word of God." Lagi emphatically nodded, responding, "true."

Further refining the topic for the evening preaching, the pastor stated, "He (Jesus) came to set us free from the power of Satan and from disease and from all sickness," to which the audience responded "hallelujah" and "*amene*" (amen). Anthropomorphizing the spirits, he said, "Our discussion is on demons; it is amazing what is happening because of the harassment of these guys."[1] These demons come in the form of alcohol, drugs, marijuana, and food, taunting people with them: "I got the smokers. I got the marijuana smokers. I have you here with food." Linking illicit substances and food, the pastor framed the problem of diet as a problem of addiction. Being addicted to food meant, the pastor said, that you "overeat, eat, eat, after you cannot move. . . . After, you cannot bend down like this." As he knelt, the congregation laughed. Demons, according to this logic, were addictions or sicknesses, collapsing spirit with body. Some sicknesses, by contrast, especially suka and toto, were "caused because you do not take care of your body." These sicknesses required those living with them to "obey what the doctor is telling you." But instead, many "still eat" after "being told." Adding levity to the sermon, he raised an eyebrow and asked, "Are you doing what the doctor tells you to do?" After some time of laughter and chatter, he continued, "but there is also a time when you will not be able to do anything unless you are delivered." This led me to wonder how congregants were to know the difference.

These kinds of scenes, across clinic and church, don't match neatly onto globally circulating stories about the "obesity epidemic," which is largely represented as a crisis of individual will (Saguy and Riley 2005; Saguy and Almeling 2008; Jutel 2009; Sanabria 2016). Instead, medical practitioners and pastors alike highlighted how individuals were located within social contexts that made individual responsibility difficult to assess. Physicians and nurses endeavored to make their patients accountable for health while also empathizing with the everyday pressures to eat and give resources to family members—things they experienced as well. Pentecostals were not immune to this endemic approach; they also encountered doctors, media, and public health campaigns that stressed individual responsibility. However, as the pastor made clear, they often maintained that, yes, individual responsibility was a factor in some cases, but other cases, and perhaps most, were *really* (undetected) problems of the spirit. One pastor even said, "the doctors call them one thing, but they are all demons." By extending the logic of demons to materials like food and fat, Pentecostals mitigated individual responsibility by looking to the contexts in which food and fat became dangerous.

Paul Rabinow (2005) argues that biological scientific discourses—ways of knowing the body and populations—have come to form the basis of sociality. Writing about the Human Genome Initiative, he suggested that scientific technologies that make nature knowable in turn make it changeable—as in detecting risk for genetic disorders, for example. In making nature changeable, scientific technologies make the cultural choices behind the use of those technologies seem natural. He calls this biosociality, where "nature will be known and remade through technique and will finally become artificial, just as culture becomes natural" (Rabinow 2005, 99). As a result, identity and emerging forms of relationships become rooted in biological or genetic conditions. For example, neurofibromatosis groups emerge to rally behind raising money for research or modifying home environments to enhance livability (Rabinow 2005, 102).

Susan Reynolds Whyte asks, "How and when do specific situated concerns move some social actors, but not others, to think and act in terms of health?" (2009, 6). In this book, I ask this question with a slight revision: how and when do specific situated concerns move some actors to use religious knowledge and related notions of spirituality to think and act in terms of health? In a context where biomedicine individualized risk, and public health efforts focused on creating a community that rallied around diet and exercise, Pentecostal Christianity provided a set of globalized practices and ideologies that anchored experiences of individual suffering and population-wide change in spiritual health. By this I mean that Christians naturalized biomedical and public health lifestyle discourses by incorporating the logic of metabolism into faith practices. The metaphor of metabolism positioned the body as an interface between God, relationships, and environments. When Pentecostals translated "eat less, exercise more" into spiritual terms, they focused on the implicit social assumptions of lifestyle discourses—individual control of diet, time, and body. They focused their attention on shaping the environment to allow for lifestyle changes to emerge from living a Christian life, creating the Kingdom of God in their own households. While making individualized change often seemed impossible, by reinterpreting biomedical assumptions through a Christian lens, these became actionable. Integrating scientific theories of cardiometabolic etiologies into religious practices for individual transformation filled the gaps left by biomedical and public health models—that is, the multiple meanings of fat, the role of wealth and poverty, and the problem of stillness.

Across Samoa, people negotiated how to eat well and demonstrate their generosity, love, and commitment to family while, as they were learning from their doctors and nurses, not jeopardizing their individual health. Pentecostals, in particular, had a clear framework from which to discern whether food, fat, and fitness posed a risk to health or were evidence of wellness. Thus, I take Pentecostal perspectives on these materials as a vivid expression of the tensions that many Samoans (not only Pentecostals) experienced around the emergence of population-wide disease—that is, the materials that once indexed wellness now also indexed sickness. Instead of straightforward valorizations of food and fat, as the literature on the health transitions might suggest, I saw ambivalence and anxiety about reciprocity and community obligation communicated through discussions of these materials. While ambiguity around the meaning of health is often left out of the discussion of the emergence of cardiometabolic disorders worldwide, this literature increasingly demonstrates the ways in which individual responsibility for cardiometabolic health is a Euro-American ideology (Crawford 2006; McNaughton 2011; Greenhalgh 2015). This ideology does not reflect how the emergence of these disorders reflects the complex interactions of social relationships, ecological patterns, and political environments in distributing risk for cardiometabolic disorders. Macro-level changes associated with urbanization, migration, and a changing food environment have all contributed to the globalization of cardiometabolic disorders, the topic I turn to next.

## THE GLOBALIZATION OF CARDIOMETABOLIC DISORDERS

In 2014, 422 million people worldwide were estimated to be living with diabetes, a near fourfold increase in thirty-five years (NCD Risk Factor Collaboration 2016).

According to the World Health Organization, over a third of the world's population is overweight or obese, and, already in 2008, 80 percent of all deaths from noncommunicable diseases (NCDs) occurred in low- and middle-income countries (Brewis 2011, 7). This global rise in diabetes and other cardiometabolic disorders reflects changes in the global economy, as these disorders are associated with urbanization, industrialization, and the growth of multinational corporations, all of which have contributed to rises in social inequalities worldwide (The Lancet 2016; Du et al. 2004). These global trends make the use of the World Bank distinction between low-, middle-, and high-income nations useful, but rough, categories for tracking the complex relationships between epidemiological, social, and economic change. Cardiometabolic disorders have been labeled diseases of "modernization" because of the ways they emerge in conjunction with increases in stress, psychological suffering, and changing social networks related to economic and social change (Mendenhall 2012; McGarvey and Baker 1979; Stunkard and Sørensen 1993; Zimmet, Alberti, and Shaw 2001; Lieberman 2003; McGarvey et al. 1989). In this way, social and economic changes predict the emergence of these disorders. For example, diabetes and obesity are the most rapidly rising in middle-income countries, such as China and India, reflecting the rapidity of social and economic changes related to further integration into global markets, including increased salaried labor, decreased physical activity, and increased consumption of processed foods (Monteiro et al. 2004). This is also true of low-income countries where "development" is thought to be a predictor of cardiometabolic disorders, not because these disorders are what was initially referred to as "diseases of affluence," but because with economic development, inequalities also increase, compacting local hierarchies while introducing new power dimensions. One clear example of how these so-called diseases of affluences are really diseases of inequalities is evidenced by the presence of the dual burden of malnutrition and overnutrition in these low-income countries (Jehn and Brewis 2009; Doaks et al. 2002). In these cases, the emergence of overweight and obesity is linked to abundance in processed foods and a related decrease in consumption of micronutrients, resulting in both over- and undernutrition (for an overview, see Tzioumis and Adair 2014).

Some scholars have used the concept of health transitions to talk about shifts in nutrition (e.g., the shift to a diet high in fats, sugar, and refined foods with corollary decreases in fiber consumption and decreases in physical activity) and epidemiology (e.g., the shift from a pattern of high frequency of acute infectious disease to one of chronic NCD) to explain global trends in rising body sizes and related diseases (Omran 1971; Popkin and Gordon-Larsen 2004; Popkin, Adair, and Ng 2012; Popkin 1994). This transition was predated by another rapid transition, the first health transition, studied by archaeologists and physical anthropologists, who have determined that there was a rapid rise in infectious disease during the Neolithic period related to climate and population changes (for an overview, see Manderson 2016). The emergence of infectious disease was largely related to shifts in social organization resulting from changing economic activities from nomadic hunting to sedentary agriculture and the domestication of animals. Even further, as populations moved, so did diseases, following shipping and commercial trading routes. The second health transition, which is associated with the decline of infectious disease, is linked to the rise in public health, regular water access, sanitation, vaccination, and other kinds of antimicrobial treatments (McKeown 1976). The emergence of NCDs reflects improved life expectancy and labor, diet, and physical activity changes. Though at the population level, there have been shifts in the prevalence of communicable to noncommunicable disease; one has not replaced the other. The emergence of HIV in the 1980s makes this particularly clear, as antiretrovirals make this communicable disease a chronic disease. Likewise, the emergence of SARS or avian flu shows how infectious disease and chronic lifestyle disease coexist (see Whyte 2012; Singer 2009; Fidler 2004). Another example that affects Samoa is that of skin ulcers related to unmanaged diabetes, which, when infected, can lead to amputation or death—showing how communicable and noncommunicable diseases become entwined in the experiences of sick persons.

Just as the health transition concept has been complicated to reflect the co-existence of communicable and noncommunicable diseases, obesity in developing countries was initially associated with the elite, but as national GDPs increase, the distribution of obesity becomes a problem of the poor (Wilkinson and Pickett 2010; Mahoney 2015). While obesity was initially associated with urban, educated women, reflecting a shift to sedentary labor and consumption of processed foods, it is increasingly impacting less educated women, reflecting the increased consumption of inexpensive, energy-dense foods and decreased walkability in residential areas (Diez Roux and Mair, 2010; Li et al., 2009). Among the poor in low- and middle-income nations, food scarcity and high-activity patterns, once "protective" factors against obesity, have now decreased, so even among the poor, there is now greater risk for obesity. These factors, compounded with lower levels of education, public infrastructure, and health knowledge, are associated with greater difficulty in acquiring less energy-dense foods, which are often more expensive (Peña and Bacallao 2000; Hojjat and Hojjat 2017; Wells et al. 2012; Swinburn et al. 2011). Increased wealth is also associated with greater opportunity for leisure time and related recreational exercise. This conventional theoretical explanation for the emergence of obesity in low-income countries suggests that economic deprivation leads to food choices that increase energy intake of negative nutrients. However, longitudinal studies show the opposite—that with resource decline, population body mass index declines or decelerates (see Hruschka 2012). For example, during the recent U.S. recession, women's obesity declined across income groups (Hruschka 2012).

Anthropological perspectives on health transitions highlight that seemingly straightforward changes from infectious disease to so-called lifestyle illnesses are always shaped by economic, social, and cultural context. The economic context is particularly clear, for example, in Korsae, Micronesia, where high rates of NCDs reflect a change in economy from subsistence production to a wage-based economy (Cassels 2006). This change limited the amount of time people had to garden and fish and, therefore, increased their dependence on tinned fish (Brownell and Yach 2006). Among Aboriginal communities in Australia, family needs often impede individual efforts to change diets, highlighting the social context of these disorders (Schwarz 2010; Dussart 2009, 2010; Saethre 2013). Finally, highlighting cultural context, people in Xela, Guatemala, often choose between foods in ways that reflect multiple models of health. People with hypertension may refuse vegetables because of the fear of pesticides, while people with diabetes may add iron-fortified sugar to their coffee for the vitamins (Yates-Doerr 2015). These brief examples show how contexts matter in ways that complicate the initial characterizations of the health transition in a linear way, where economic development is accompanied by the distribution of disease because these distributions are further shaped by local contexts.

Certain nations and groups of people have also become the research epitome of epidemiological change—Pacific Islanders and Native Americans in North America, for instance—because of the rapidity of these trends (Ferrerira, Leal, and Lang 2006; Baker, Hanna, and Baker 1986; Olson 2001). On a global scale, over 50 percent of indigenous adults—defined here as First Peoples in Canada, the Americas, the Pacific Islands, New Zealand, Australia, Asia, and Africa—have type 2 diabetes (Harris et al. 2017). The American Diabetes Association reports that American Indians and Alaska Natives have the highest prevalence of diabetes in the United States at 16 percent (American Diabetes Association 2017), and cardiometabolic disorders are in the top five leading causes of death among Native Americans (Heron 2016). The rapid rise in these disorders is clear in the following estimate: from 1994 to 2004, rates of diabetes among Native Americans rose 68 percent (American Diabetes Association 2017). As recently as 2015, the Centers for Disease Control and Prevention estimated that, among American Indians in the Southwest, the prevalence of diabetes is 22 percent (Centers for Disease Control and Prevention 2017).

One of the best-documented cases of the emergence of diabetes, building on nearly forty years of National Institutes of Health clinical research, is among Pima people living at Gila River (Smith-Morris 2007). It has become impossible to separate this history of research from the experiences of diabetes among Pima people; as Carolyn Smith-Morris notes, "the investigation itself" has become "part of the Pima pathology" (2006, 6; 2007). Among Pima people, the political and economic factors that have influenced the emergence of diabetes began in the 1800s with colonization. By the late nineteenth century, Pima farms had no water, and their eventual loss of arable land left them dependent on the federal government for food (Smith-Morris 2006). Pima people, as with other Native Americans, face what Dennis Wiedman (2012) calls "chronicities of modernity"—that is, chronic diseases that result from the physical containment of the body when reservations are created, which ultimately limit physical activity while leading to overnutrition and chronic stress. Social, ecological, and economic changes involved with colonialism, such as the shift from agriculture to a cash economy, related shifts from community-produced foods to mass processed foods, and changes in transportation are all implicated. In addition, there have been changes in physical activity from reduced agriculture, as well as overnutrition, and undernutrition from changes in diet, and chronic stress related to colonization. Technological changes like the introduction of refrigerators and electric and gas cooking allowed people to shift from wood fires to electric or gas cooking, which introduced the culinary possibility of frying food. Refrigerators also reduced the need to share food within social networks, as it became possible to preserve and save food for individuals (for similar factors impacting Samoa, see Macpherson and Macpherson 2009, 168).

The anthropology of diabetes has brought to the fore of scholarly attention the importance of chronic and extreme psychosocial stress from forced assimilation and rapid integration into the global economy, and extreme inequalities flowing from this (Garro 1995; Scheder 1988; Rock 2003; Schoenberg et al. 2005; Manderson and Kokanovic 2009; Mendenhall et al. 2012a, 2012b; Montesi 2017; for a review, see Ferzacca 2012). As access to material goods changed, so too did the symbolic dimensions of prestige, shaping how social identities were expressed—thereby showing how rapid epidemiological change is as much a matter of calories as the capacity to access symbolic materials, land, and relationships. This combination of changing materiality and the meaning of that materiality creates environments that can be chronically stressful. This is directly connected to the emergence of cardiometabolic disorders. William Dressler and James Bindon (2000) demonstrate how chronic stress, evidenced by rises in stress hormones, results from a mismatch between life expectations and life chances, economic insecurity and high cost of living, and a lack of sense of control and related disintegration of social support, which places people at higher risk of developing diabetes (for evidence from Samoa, see also Bindon, Crews, and Dressler 1991; Bindon et al. 1997; Janes 1990; McDade 2001, 2002). Emily Mendenhall (2012) has described the emergence of diabetes among Mexican migrant women as the VIDDA (violence, migration-related stress, depression, diabetes, and domestic abuse) syndemic. She uses a syndemic framework to describe "situations in which adverse social conditions, such as poverty and oppressive social relationships, stress a population, weaken its natural defenses, and expose it to a cluster of interacting diseases" (2012, 13; Weaver and Mendenhall 2014).

The social suffering associated with both risk for cardiometabolic disorders and the experience of living with cardiometabolic disorders is compounded by the further racialization of populations through the research process. Indigenous populations in Oceania and North America have served as "natural experiments" or "living laboratories" for understanding rapid social change, positioning people as research "subjects" first and foremost. The initial framing of the emergence of chronic disease was as a "mismatch disease," suggesting that the bodies of indigenous peoples were not modern enough for the changing social world (Klingle 2015). These teleological frameworks reproduce Euro-American narratives about the inappropriate fit of indigenous peoples with modernity, thereby normalizing the unequal distribution of suffering and disease (see Yates-Doerr 2015). Others, like Michael Montoya (2011), look to the ways that diabetes research is an ideological project, reproducing *and* resisting the naturalization of diabetes with Mexican-ness through the dehistoricizing of diabetes etiologies.

## OBESITY IN OCEANIA

The search for a genetic cause of obesity has also shaped research in Oceania, increasingly naturalizing the "Obese Samoan." The historical legacy of food shortage has been used to hypothesize that islanders have a greater genetic predisposition to gain weight because of their so-called thrifty gene (Neel 1962; McGarvey 1995; cf. Fee 2006). More recently, long-time Samoa researcher Stephen McGarvey, with Nicola Hawley and colleagues, found a genetic variant among Samoans that increased the risk of becoming overweight or obese (Minster et al. 2016). The authors of this work are clear to point out, however, that this variant does not predetermine who will become overweight or obese, and more than 55 percent of Samoans do not have the genetic variant associated with increased risk. Other social, political, and economic factors also play a part.

The Pacific Islands bear a particularly high burden of cardiometabolic disorders, and the World Bank estimates that 70 percent or more of all deaths in the Pacific Islands are related to NCDs (Anderson 2013). Between 1980 and 2010, of all regions in the world, countries in Oceania had the greatest increase in body mass index (Finucane et al. 2011). Life expectancy has actually fallen in places like Tonga as a result (Anderson 2013). In Samoa, the rapid rise in cardiometabolic disorders is particularly striking and evident in the following statistical estimates: between 1978 and 1991, obesity increased in males by 297 percent and in females by 115 percent in rural Samoa (Hodge et al. 1994). Recent statistics suggest that over 66 percent of the Samoan population is obese (Hawley et al. 2014). The total prevalence of overweight and obesity among females was 93.5 percent and 86.5 percent for men (Hawley et al. 2014). While among women, age did not significantly affect the prevalence of overweight and obesity, among men, overweight and obesity was more prevalent in older age (Hawley et al. 2014). Regarding hypertension, women are less likely than men to be affected (31.7 percent versus 36.7 percent), while the prevalence of diabetes is equivalent (17.8 percent [females] versus 16.4 percent [males]) (Hawley et al. 2014). There is also significant regional variation, with urban areas being associated with higher risk of obesity and diabetes, reflecting labor and dietary differences between urban and rural populations (Hawley et al. 2014; Barnes et al. 2010). These macroassessments bear out the ways that social histories of colonization—that is, the ways that histories of contact have influenced migration, urbanization, and food availability—have all contributed to the rapid rise of these disorders (see McLennan and Ulijaszek 2015a, 2015b).

Migration is a rite of passage for young Samoan people, creating a pattern of leaving the islands with the intention to return later with resources like cash, clothes, food, and prestige (Lilomaiava-Doktor 2009; Va'a 2001; for examples from the region, see also Alexeyeff 2013; Lee and Francis 2009; Lee 2003; Ka'ili 2005). Samoans and many other Pacific Islanders have large diaspora communities in places like the United States, New Zealand, and Australia, where they are also found to have high rates of overweight, obesity, and cardiometabolic disorders. For example, Samoan-born people in Queensland, Australia, were seven times as likely to be hospitalized for diabetes-related complications than the general Queensland population (Queensland Government 2011). This suggests that migration, with changed labor patterns, changed diets, and significant barriers to healthcare, including cost or lack of transport, exacerbates these disorders. Migrants also face new stresses related to the demands of maintaining family relations—mostly through remittances—while living abroad (Capstick et al. 2009; Janes 1990; Brown and Ahlburg 1999; McGarvey and Seiden 2010). These remittances, and the new ideals that returned migrants develop around economic opportunity and change, make them "agents of modernization," which scholars link to new preferences for and the ability to purchase imported foods as well as to have the means to purchase those foods with remittances (Ulijaszek 2005).

Urbanization has also encouraged Samoans to move away from agricultural labor, which can be very physically demanding, to more sedentary activities. This move away from agricultural labor is derived from lack of land in urban areas as well as increased opportunities for wage and salary labor associated with sedentary jobs.[2] Additionally, people tend to drive cars more often and use public transport rather than walk. By 2020, the Asian Development Bank (2014) estimates that more than one-half of the population of the Pacific Islands will live and work in towns, which suggests that cardiometabolic disorders will only increase. The epidemiology of cardiometabolic disorders also reflects this trend where, in Samoa, the more urban the population—that is, those who live in Apia and surrounding villages—the higher the rates of cardiometabolic disorders. Part of the reason that urban communities have higher rates of cardiometabolic disorders is that people tend to continue to eat large meals on Sundays, as well as during fa'alavelave, but do not have the same physical activity demands associated with rural living, which tends to counterbalance periodic feasting. In a study as early as 1982, Hodge and colleagues (1994) found that urban residents consumed fewer calories throughout the week than those living in the rural villages, but they consumed equal amounts on the weekends, an average of 5,930 calories per day compared to the 5,940 calories consumed by rural villagers. However, urban residents did not engage in physical activity during the week to offset weekend consumption.

Another macro change related to the emergence of these disorders is global changes in food availability and prices. The small size of the island populations, and their limited agricultural productive capacity due to the relatively small amount of arable land and distance from major markets, makes most island nations dependent on imported foods while simultaneously powerless in international trade policy negotiations (McLennan and Ulijaszek 2015a, 2015b; see also Pollock 1986). This context of trade influences food choices more than food preferences and knowledge of nutritional value, as local, low-fat sources of proteins, such as fish, often cost up to 50 percent more than imported fatty meats (for a study in Tonga, see Evans et al. 2001; see also Choy et al. 2017). In Samoa, there has been a rapid rise in the availability of fat from poultry, mutton, and vegetable oil, which can be linked to the globalization of food production as well as decreases in trade regulations, making imported foods relatively cheap (Seiden et al. 2012; Errington and Gewertz 2008; Gewertz and Errington 2007, 2010; Keighley et al. 2007). Population-wide dietary changes were thus foreshadowed by changes to the regulations of the importation of poultry, pork, and rice, all of which were limited until the mid-1970s—the same time that cardiometabolic disorders begin to rise (Seiden et al. 2012, 293). Food aid has also contributed to dietary change, as cereals, including rice, are imported to address food shortages due to natural disasters like cyclones or taro blight and then become household staples (Galanis et al. 1999; see also Wang 2017).

As described above, cardiometabolic disorders clearly demonstrate how population-wide health is impacted by a changing global economy, where macro-level trends in urbanization, migration, and food availability and diet impact individuals, communities, and populations. I draw from critical medical anthropology to add to this scholarly theory of health transitions by bringing forward places and stories that highlight Samoan perspectives on the ways that inequalities shape the distribution of risk. In particular, I highlight how cultural context matters in determining when materials like food, fat, and fitness were thought to be dangerous or beneficial to health. Critical medical anthropology frameworks seek to contextualize health, illness, and suffering within political and economic context, accounting for the historical emergence of health inequities as they are tied to global capitalism (see Baer, Singer, and Johnsen 1986; Singer et al. 1992). These broader political and economic forces "pattern human relationships, shape social behaviors, condition collective experiences, reorder local ecologies, and situate cultural meanings" (Baer, Singer, and Susser 2003, 43). In Samoa, at the micro level, social and economic changes can be seen in how family relations unfold over increasingly distant spaces—between village and the urban center, for instance—and over national boundaries—as in between Samoa and the diaspora. Changes in food availability have shifted the material ways that relatedness is expressed—through cash, tinned meats, and bolts of fabric instead of the taro, local chicken, and fine mats of previous generations. A can of Coke or a bottle of red wine now replaces the coconut that would be served to matai during fa'alavelave. These changes create contradictions in everyday life around the meanings of food, fat, and fitness, which are essential both to expand the social history of epidemiological change and to understand how to more effectively address prevention efforts. Macrotheoretical models that link wealth, body positivity, and physical activity levels to emerging rates of cardiometabolic disorders are important tools for understanding population change; however, these trends tell us little about the experience of the social change that has propelled the epidemiological change. In the remainder of this chapter, I explore four cultural discourses that highlight contradictions in biomedical etiologies for cardiometabolic disorders, making spiritual health a common-sense frame for dealing with moral ambiguity. These include the following contradictions: (1) wealth and poverty are associated with cardiometabolic risk; (2) fat can mean power, generosity, and generativity, *and* laziness, sickness, and moral corruption; (3) foods that have historically created well-being now make people sick; and, finally, (4) health promotion situates fa'asamoa as both the source of risk and the source of healthy behaviors.

## WEALTH AND POVERTY

In a joking tone, poking fun at what he thought was a backward, or cultural, point of view, one physician said, "You know the people they think, if you are fat, you are wealthy." Another took this idea one step further and reflected on how changing health outcomes was about changing culture: "I think, creating a whole shift in mentality about our relationship with food and what our definition is of wealth and beauty. Our definition of wealth does not necessarily have to be, we don't necessarily have to demonstrate wealth through having so much food." Just as scholars are tracking the complex relationships between wealth and obesity, Samoans were concerned with understanding when wealth or poverty both created risk for developing cardiometabolic disorders. On the one hand, poor people were the sickest. They didn't have the money to purchase "healthy foods" like vegetables, nor did they have the resources to seek out healthcare when needed. They were also thought to sacrifice their own nutritional needs to provide gifts to pastors and other community leaders, which was exacerbated by the experience of ever-increasing demands for cash. The wealthy and powerful, on the other hand, were thought to get sick because they were able to eat without limits or labor, as their communities provided only their best (fatty, salty, and sweet) foods as symbols of their generosity and respect. These prototypes are polar opposites in a Samoan worldview, and yet they were both thought to suffer the same disorders. This can be explained by thinking of how food and fat are more than biological materials, but also materials that move in a moral economy. While it is easy to imagine reciprocity as the movement of gifts between people, reciprocity is also a process of creating bodies through the capacities of those gifts. Cash and food are gifts of potentiality—they grow relationships and they grow bodies. The first anthropological paper on obesity emphasizes this potentiality as evidence by common sayings like these: "We shall be glad, we shall eat until we vomit," from the Trobriand Islands, or "We shall eat until our bellies swell out and we can no longer stand," a saying from South Africa (Powdermaker 1960, 286). Similarly, in Samoa, after attending a wedding, people will ask about the food. To say there wasn't much food is a way to insult the hosting families.

To understand the ways that the poor and the wealthy were thought to be sick—the poor because they are vulnerable and the wealthy because they are powerful—is to understand that families remain "a foundation of Samoan society" as they form "microeconomies that hold and manage the family estate, which typically comprises agricultural land and house sites in a village, and periodically, raise and invest funds usually in sociopolitical activity on behalf of their members" (Macpherson and Macpherson 2009, 13). Matai are divided into two categories: *ali'i* (chiefs) and *tulafale* (orators). Orators speak for ali'i, revealing a distributed power where quiet stillness is emblematic of high chiefs and their power. The political system is also deeply tied to kinship because only matai can serve in the National Legislative Assembly. Universal suffrage was extended in 1990, as before this, only matai could vote. Families are managed by matai who are given their titles for their abilities to serve their family. They govern the village through participation in the *fono* (village council) (Macpherson and Macpherson 2009, 13), frequently organizing capital fundraising projects to build or rebuild churches and schools, access roads to plantations, or support village beautification.[3] These projects are a way for families and villages to compete in order to "raise the name" or "develop" the village, which "reinforces both the villages' and the families' collective identities, and indirectly, their codependence" (Macpherson and Macpherson 2009, 15). Individuals exchange their labor, and the fruits of that labor like food and fine mats, for land rights and protection, which are material expressions of central Samoan values like *tautua* (service), *alofa* (generosity/ love), and *fa'aaloalo* (respect). However, today it is also essential for family members to have access to cash in order to fully participate in family-building activities. In tune with this change, I often heard statements like, "We used to be strong; now we have all these sicknesses." When I would ask why, people focused on changing diets and the cost of food: "Everything costs money now." This pressure to give cash was not just around ritual exchange but also for daily expenses— school fees, medical costs, church donations, and cellphone credit—that individuals often cannot meet with their own resources.

Another way anxieties about reciprocity were expressed was by blaming the poor for their sickness. Mata'afa Keni Lesa (2012a), an editorial writer for the Samoan daily newspaper, the *Samoa Observer,* makes this clear: "The point is that, if we want a healthier Samoa, the change has to come from within. It is about changing mindsets, reversing bad habits, and telling ourselves that what we have here in Samoa is perfectly fine for us and our health." The author suggests that individuals need to change their behaviors—"reversing their bad habits"—and as with health professionals, he jumps from focusing on poverty to culture. The implicit statement here is that people have access to "healthy" foods from their subsistence gardens, but they choose the "unhealthy" foods associated with prestige whenever possible—another shorthand way to critique culture. When Lesa writes that Samoans need to tell themselves "what we have here in Samoa is perfectly fine," he is talking about the perceived misplaced desire, among mostly the poor, for imported, expensive foods. The poor were thought to be fat not only because they give away their best resources—food and cash—but also because they traded in the foods they grow on their own land, ostensibly "healthy" and "free," for purchasable foods that are thought to be "unhealthy" and "expensive." This was a widely circulating stereotype that Lesa adds to when he writes, "I have a friend who used to come every Saturday to sell his taro and bananas in the old market. He would stand or sit in the sun and rain till his produce was sold, then got in a taxi, bought his beers and packets of cigarettes, went home, and got wasted. He is now an ill man, frequents the hospital, living with NCDs" (2012a).

Here, poor and uneducated people are "careless" about their health, making "small choices" that are "sweet for the taste buds but extremely sour for the poor intestines" (Lesa 2012a). More critically, Lesa draws attention to how indigenous foods, such as banana and mango, "go to waste on the trees" as Samoans aim to eat imported foods with higher prestige, such as expensive New Zealand apples or "hard biscuits and lollies that wreak havoc on our teeth" (2012a). This echoes the widely circulating critique of poor farmers or fishermen who sell their agricultural goods or fish only to purchase tinned fish, imported meat, or rice—the more prestigious products that are pictured as expensive and unhealthy alternatives to the "more nutritious" indigenous and "free" foods (Hardin and Kwauk 2015, 524).

This cash-poverty narrative contrasts the ways that community leaders like pastors, matai, and government leaders were thought to get fat and sick from the foods they ate and received from others. One woman contrasted her grandfather, who was a pastor, as thin and sunburned from laboring on his own land, catching his own fish, to her current village pastor who was a "big, lazy man" (Macpherson and Macpherson 2009, 137). This pastor was the recipient of myriad gifts—the village paid for his house, food, and petrol in addition to a monthly stipend. She thought he stored all the food gifts the congregation gave to him in his "big freezer" to give to his own family, rather than to give it back to the congregation

(Macpherson and Macpherson 2009, 137). One pastor from my AOG church was extolled for working with a small herd of cattle on his own land during the week. These kinds of stories show how many Samoans understand cardiometabolic disorders in deeply contextual ways—not all fat is the same, it is more than the metrics of weight, height, and calories, and accumulation methods matter in creating sickness.

These simultaneous explanations that link poverty and wealth with the rapid rise in cardiometabolic disorders reflect a paradox in research on global obesity. In low-income countries, men, women, and children with higher socioeconomic status are more likely to be overweight, while in high-income countries, the reverse is true (Sobal and Stunkard 1989; McLaren 2007). In middle-income countries, inequalities, urbanization, and poverty rise in sync with obesity (see Brewis 2011, 64). Samoa is one case where there is rapid economic change—recently "graduating" from the least developed countries list to a small group of countries classified as developing in 2014 (see UN-OHRLLS 2017)—making it difficult to discern whether being wealthy or poor puts one at a greater risk for developing cardiometabolic disorders. This paradox—that both wealthy and poor people are sick—is not a contradiction as much as spiritual evidence for Pentecostals that reciprocity is not working to everyone's advantage, at least not in the way that was imagined it should.

## STRONG LARGE BODIES, SICK OBESE BODIES

Scholars have a long history of investigating body image, body size, and beauty ideals (for a review, see Gremillion 2005; see also Anderson-Fye and Brewis 2017). Until recently, this attention tended to be limited to a framework that suggests that cultures view fat in one of three ways—positively, neutrally, or negatively (see Hardin 2015b). Accordingly, Euro-American cultures tend to be represented as fat loathing, while non-European cultures—in Africa, Latin America, Oceania—tend to be represented as fat positive.[4] Fat negativity and positivity, however, often coexist (see Lupton 2013). For example, African American women tend to be represented in this research as fat positive, yet ethnography suggests that this positivity is not so straightforward (McClure 2017). Young black women might value "curves" while also articulating fat stigma, therefore complicating the idea that African American women are fat positive and at higher risk for obesity as a result.[5] In research about obesity in Oceania, fat positivity is considered a risk factor for obesity, entrenching the idea that, when fat is not repudiated, it must be risky to health.[6]

To complicate matters, fat stigma, notions of obesity as disease, and ideas of fat as reflecting personal and social failing have spread as rates of obesity also rise globally (Brewis et al. 2011). Anne Becker (2004), in her work in Fiji, found with the introduction of television came a newfound desire for thinner, fitter bodies among young adolescent girls, reflecting their active construction of their own identities in a rapidly changing global economy—thinner, fitter bodies could lead to better jobs and allow them to fit into a new social environment. Eileen Anderson-Fye (2004) similarly found that, among young women in Belize, a desire for a thinner body reflected desires for economic opportunities in the tourism industry, rather than a personal desire to be thin. Studies like these show both the globalization of fat stigma and the importance of looking to context to understand how the meaning of fat is multivalent.

One way to begin to unpack how fat can have multiple meanings, both cross-culturally and within particular contexts, is to think about the relationship between body and care. In Fiji, for example, the body "reflects the achievements of its caretakers," where "crafting" the body was the "province of the community rather than the self" (Becker 1995, 56). In this context, fatness indicated community wellness, and by extension, excess fat was considered negative because it restricted an individual's ability to contribute to community. References to hunger or satiety are, therefore, "metacommunication" about embodied care (Becker 1995, 67). In Samoa, discussions about fat, as well as hunger and satiety, were often discussions about relationships. Lesa's editorials are helpful here as well. He writes, "Have you ever undertaken one of those weight loss challenges where you've shed a few kilos only to be told by your mother that you look rather sick?" (2012a). In fact, he writes, "This is a country where in some cases they say the bigger, the better." I found that in everyday life, calling someone fat was not ordinarily an insult, as joking and teasing about body size was quite common. I learned this when my research assistant commented on a photo of me on social media, which had been taken the year before I started fieldwork. After some posts from others, she wrote, "Wow u look so fat . . . lol." After feeling a bit of discomfort about the comment, when I met up with her later, I asked her about it. She told me she thought I looked quite happy, probably because I was home with my family. She then asked me if I missed them. My weight loss indexed my distance from my family. Perhaps I wasn't eating enough and she worried I was getting sick. This kind of mundane teasing about fat was a way to show she cared.

Stillness also demonstrates care. As an embodied mode of wellness and dignity, to be still was to indicate status (e.g., to be served) and the strength of the family's capacity to serve. Typically, as Samoan people age, they engage in less and less physical activity, encouraging those beneath them in household hierarchies to do the chores and agricultural labor. Physical activity patterns are also gendered; most explained that, once child rearing begins, men tend to become less active, including reduced plantation labor and leisure activities of rugby. After they have had children, women tend to become stationary and do less demanding chores. Young women, with or without children, often do not have the opportunity for sport-based leisure activities either (Kwauk 2014a). In formal contexts, the still-sitting matai embodies dignity as the orator communicates for him. The matai is served, his needs anticipated by others. Even Tui Atua Tupua Tamasese Efi, the Samoan Head of State, was criticized for jogging in shorts and t-shirt, and matai are sometimes advised by their family members at fa'alavelave to sit quietly, observing everyone else rushing around, working (Schoeffel, personal communication). The dignity of the *taupou* (village maiden) is similarly communicated through controlled movement. She dances gracefully, with delicately choreographed hand movements; her brother wildly dances, slaps his chest, and lies on the floor as she elegantly raises a foot and places it on his back (see also Alexeyeff 2009). Physical activity is thus humorous, and often associated with young men.[7] In each of these examples, stillness and movement introduce a world of meaning about age, sexuality, and status. Conversely, physical activity (i.e., walking, jogging, or running) could introduce ridicule or shame, as these activities draw attention to the body and disrupt the village landscape of peacefulness. This dignity—in body and place—became clear to me one afternoon as I sat on the front porch at one of my household field sites. I hardly noticed as some village children began to play in front of the house, but, within minutes, my adopted mother appeared, scolding the children for not acting "respectfully" and "acting like animals." My adopted sister would later explain to me that the children were not to play in front of the house because she was a matai, and even the space of her house should exude dignity and so be reserved for quietness.

The dignity of quietness and stillness stood in contrast to widely popular Polynesian Zumba that was proliferating during my fieldwork. Every day, women gathered to dance with other women for their health and explicitly to lose weight. Classes were held in private gyms or national sports facilities, and for a fee, you could dance with up to fifty other women. The instructors adapted dance aerobics and Zumba instruction with Polynesian dance movements and rhythms. In these largely urban female spaces, women could reformulate their expressions of dignity by using humor to create lively environments for physical activity. The classes attracted women in part because of the biblical advertisements, calling interested people to "come as they are." These factors made physical activity a source of cultural and religious pride, within a deeply female and positive domain, where women could dance to be physical active—they could sweat, push each other and themselves, all the while joking and teasing one another. The women valued the use of traditional dance and music, prayer, and the experience of family inclusiveness—that is, the leadership was community oriented (see Heard et al. 2016). The gendering of the space in addition to its religious framing and culturally explicitly Polynesian-ness made this activity appropriate and valued for urban women of all ages. Physical activities thus encompass a wide range of practices and meanings. While urban, and wealthy, men and women created a demand for gyms and fitness classes ranging from Zumba to spin to circuit weight lifting, physical activity in villages revolved around the labor of fulfilling obligations and feeding one's family. The opportunity, or burden, of physical activities was shaped by status, age, and gender, fashioning how one could, and should, use the body in public spaces.

## GOOD FOOD, BAD FOR HEALTH

Sitting at a desk in front of a floral curtain, I interviewed Sefina, a nurse who was also a hospital administrator, when she told me how she really wanted to make a change in her own community, but she was consistently blocked by her peers. Sefina was the leader of the women's group at church, and when she suggested serving papaya, coconut, and mango and orange leaf tea to a group of visiting pastors, the women scoffed. How could they serve pastors the same foods that pigs eat? The group insisted on preparing heaping trays of corned beef sandwiches with milky, sugary black tea. Serving guests local fruits would have been embarrassing because these foods, especially coconut, were reserved for animals and were "free" foods. Serving these foods could indicate that the church didn't have enough money to purchase *mea lelei* (good food), or didn't respect them enough to serve them these good foods, reflecting the historical connection between "lands, food, and family (past and present)" (McMullin 2010, 13).

Eating in my households every day was a community effort, meaning almost everyone in the household contributed in some way. In my Assemblies of God household, the youngest brother would prepare the *saka*, the boiling of starches, during the week. On the weekend, he would prepare the *umu* (earth oven), with all the men in the house, which required them to wake as early as three in the morning to begin heating the rocks. The youngest brother would make coconut cream—scraping the meat from the coconut and then squeezing it out— contributing the most essential ingredient for each meal. Those who worked in town would purchase additional items like chicken or tinned fish, which the eldest daughter of the household would prepare when she returned from work. If there was no money to purchase something to eat with the starches, the matriarch would retrieve cans of corned beef, rice, or tinned fish hidden under the bed, in her locked bedroom. If this stock was low, then the household ate fruit soups, that is, papaya or banana cooked with coconut cream and tapioca pearls. While I delighted in this option, it usually made others grumble that they felt hungry. The way this family ate reflected general Samoan food categorizations where a meal required starches and some kind of other food, preferably meat, to complement the starches (see Pollock 1992).

*Mea'a'ano* are staple foods, including taro, banana, and breadfruit; these foods strengthen the body and are deeply connected to the *fanua* (the land) and the *'āiga* (the family). Mea'a'ano requires *mea lelei* (good food) to complement the starches, including fresh meat, tinned meat, *mea lololo* (fatty meat), or, more typically, tinned fish. Foods like fruits, fruit soups, and, today, sandwiches, processed snack foods, and instant noodles were eaten throughout the day but are not generally

considered essential to mealtimes nor were they considered "real" food (cf. Pollock 1985). Good foods are good in part because they carry prestige because they
are cultural objects of exchange; they create wellness by indexing social networks
that can be experienced through their consumption (cf. Becker 1995). They are
also satisfying because they are fatty or salty, or both. Good foods are also good
because they are partible. In other words, tinned meats come in cases that can be
broken down, redistributed, and consumed over a long period of time and, therefore, enter into households through ritual exchange. These foods derive their
value from their capacity to create satiety that is both about taste and the experience of the good life.

Good food, therefore, was often bad for health, which created daily struggles
for those living with cardiometabolic disorders. Just as John craved "healthy"
foods, my interlocutors from the diabetes clinic craved good foods. When interviewing in the clinic, one man explained his difficulty with changing his diet: "I can
see the piece of pork lying there and the fried chicken leg. Well, I crave it. It is
tempting you, even when I am given food cooked with vegetables that's good
because it helps with my diabetes. It is best for me." The vegetable-based options
were good for health, but not the good foods that he craved. One physician
summed up these contrasting views of foods saying, with frustration, "Well, you
see this is the irony of it. The good food is all the fatty stuff. Meanwhile, you have
fruit rotting on the trees." Some of my clinic research participants were often left
with the choice of not eating or eating foods they knew were not good for health.[8]
One woman said in times when she was very stressed about money, "it's better to
eat even when it's bad food."

Those without access to labor or land were the most vulnerable to this experience (Thornton, Binns, and Kerslake 2013). Lea, a woman in her late forties, was
one such example. Her husband had died and she lived alone with her son. Instead
of insisting that her son work the plantation, which would be reasonable given
this would provide staple foods and, from the sale of crops, the family's only access
to cash, Lea insisted her son stay in school. This meant Lea, like many other
women, tended the plantation for household consumption but not for cash crop-
ping. She said, sometimes, "there is nothing; I don't know where to find food,
maybe in the ocean sometimes. Sometimes I only boil a bunch of bananas for the
whole day and night." She reassured her son, "Don't worry about a special dish.
You will always have special dishes when you have a job." This special dish refers
to the now-required accompaniment to starches, that is, meat, without which
people felt they were deprived.

Many of those who did have access to cash explained that they often gave their
available good foods to their pastor. "If I have corned beef or bananas, they go to
our pastor first," one man in his seventies explained. Another woman in her fifties said, "I am very worried when it comes to money. When there is not enough
for church things, family things, sometimes we don't have any food." Sometimes,

after families had fulfilled their obligations, "there's not really much left for food." One physician explained she knew her grandfather would often "hide his money for cultural obligations even though we didn't have any food." While these families were likely not skipping all meals because most had access to starches, sometimes there were only these starches. If additional cash was available, then meat might be purchased to complete the meal (see also Fitzgerald 1986). One physician explained, "When people have a chance to eat if they're at a wedding or a funeral and food is provided, then they will eat as much as they can." Another diabetes clinic patient said, "Whatever foods I get, that's it. If they give me pork, I eat it all." Good foods are also unevenly distributed within single households. In formal contexts, as well as many households, the elders eat first, with junior family members preparing and serving meals. After the elders, the women and small children eat, followed by the untitled men. In this arrangement, the elders, or high-status people, like pastors or matai, eat the best foods, while others eat what remains, which isn't always a lot. These daily negotiations of what to eat, where to get food, and who to share it with made eating a rather fraught everyday project, especially for those who were cash poor *and* living with cardiometabolic disorders.

## HEALTH PROMOTION

Within the last decade, the Ministry of Health (MOH) has created a new category of food, *mea'ai paleni* (literally, balanced food), in an attempt to create value around foods like fruits and vegetables. This category of food, which local and international development agencies have aggressively promoted in public health campaigns, expands what it means to eat a full meal by adding fruits and vegetables to a complementary meal of starch and meat. Yet, vegetables were also often considered "empty" and "tasteless," while fruits were often considered children's food or even "pig's food." One physician said, "The problem here in Samoa is vegetables have never been an important part of the diet. Vegetables and fruits are just filling, to just fill your belly. It's not food. The kids will eat mangos in the mango season until they are sick cause they're hungry, but it is not regarded as food. It's not part of your healthy diet, or well-being. It's just stuff your stomach until you can get a decent meal. Like, fried fish." Vegetables were often associated with imported varieties, including cabbage, lettuce, tomatoes, and apples, that were perceived to be not only expensive, but also unfulfilling (Hardin and Kwauk 2015). Their perceived expense may reflect the fact that they are considered nice but unnecessary. In fact, some vegetables, like the eggplant that I would purchase and contribute to my household dinners, would remain unused, becoming limp in the refrigerator, while other vegetables like leafy greens or cucumbers would be readily incorporated because they could be easily added to already-conceptualized meals. Meals largely consisted of soups and fried meats, so vegetables that could be added to soups made sense, but if they were not easily added, they did not change the meal.

One way that the morality of healthy eating is communicated to a Samoan medical public (i.e., those Samoans engaged with medicine, who visit the hospitals and clinics) is through health promotion posters. Various posters were widely visible across government offices, shops, and medical facilities. The posters encouraged the audience to see food differently, to think about food as made of constitutive elements: namely, fat, nutrients, sugar, etc. These constitutive parts were implicitly categorized as good (nutrients, lean meat) or bad (fat, sugar). The logic is supposed to be easy: "With the input and output established, what more is there to know?" (Yates-Doerr 2012a, 294). Viewers were intended to relearn how to choose foods based on nutritional values and rank these foods as more valuable than other foods valued for alternative reasons. In these posters, adapted for Pacific Islander audiences, common foods like fried fish, taro, coconut cream, and chips were converted into teaspoons of fat. For example, a can of Coke is equivalent to eight teaspoons of sugar and a fillet of fried fish is equivalent to nine teaspoons of fat. In contrast, a plate of three pieces of boiled taro is equivalent to zero teaspoons of fat. In another campaign, "Slash da Salt," the MOH highlights another single ingredient as an additive to be reduced. In still other posters, viewers learn how to reduce fat by preparing meat in new ways. Step one in each of these posters teaches methods for removing fat. For unprepared meats, the instruction is to remove "visible fat," while the fat in corned beef can be reduced by boiling the can and then draining the excess fat. In turn, each poster instructs the viewer to see fat as trash (step two in making healthier mutton flaps is to "throw fat away"). These posters also call for the addition of "lots of colored vegetables" in addition to "staple foods, such as taro or green banana." The instructions, therefore, aim to enhance meat and starch meals with added nutrients in the form of vegetables, not ordinarily considered a necessary component for a satisfactory meal.

The kind of cooking-as-conceptualizing illustrated in the poster renders fat excess or as waste, not as a valued element—fat that is precisely what makes these meats valuable as gifts. In fact, there are Samoan common-sense ways to divide the meat of animals. For fa'alavelave, certain cuts of meat are distributed to high-status people. But the health promotion materials sought to teach people to value meat and other foods for their nutritional components rather than by their role in building social relationships. The added value in these posters is the vegetables, because of their health-giving qualities. The targeted problem is not the food itself, but in the ways in which food is conceptualized as part of the "healthier" (read nutritionally balanced) meal. The viewer is encouraged to think about food in terms of its invisible elemental (nutritional) parts and change behaviors as a result.[9]

Public health messaging also crosses over into agricultural development in posters designed to diversify diets and agricultural products. The Nutrition Center of MOH presented at annual agricultural fairs, and in 2012, they produced a poster, "Grow and Eat Dark-Green Leafy Vegetables." At fair presentations, MOH staff would encourage farmers to grow more varieties of edible green vegetables while also educating farmers on edible greens potentially already growing on their land. These edible greens are local but not always recognized as food. My adopted sister often teased me about eating "only leaves" when I ate these varieties of greens, insisting that I must be hungry all the time as a result. Other posters focused on "Easy and Cheap Foods" that were abundant in everyday life, linking greens that grew wild or very easily to breast milk as free and easy foods. Other posters featured diagrams showing the nutrient and vitamin content of taro, coconut, banana, and banana chips. The assumption of all of these posters, and the presence of health officials at these fairs, is that poor knowledge of nutrition and plant species is interconnected and an impediment to health.

Many local health professionals also valorized local foods for their superior nutritional qualities associated with health, in contrast to imported foods. For example, one local fitness instructor sold coconuts and smoothies after her classes. She posted on Facebook a picture of two coconuts with plastic straws, with the caption, "Perfect way to refresh yourself in the islands with God's fruit." Indigenous foods—coconut, taro, banana—were also used to explain why Samoan people are *malosi* (strong). For example, as my adopted sister began to introduce solids to her six-month-old baby, her father whispered to me during our evening meal, "Samoan babies are stronger then *pālagi* (white/European) babies" precisely because the baby was beginning to eat the taro that his mother had prechewed. The logic suggests that Samoan babies eat *mea'a'ano* and not pālagi foods, and they are strong as a result. The son-in-law, noticing the commentary his father-in-law was providing, said, "The baby will be a rugby player. So he needs to eat his taro to become strong." Imported baby food was "weak food." It is not food that babies needed to become *lapo'a* (big/fat) and malosi.

This linkage between strength and starches was incorporated into public health campaigns as well. In one commercial designed for television, a scientist-type figure raps, "If you like drinking tea and eating bread, change now your butter to avocado. You have power." The scientist again encourages the viewer to replace high-fat, negative nutrients, like butter, with local alternatives. Then appears another teen boy carrying an *amo* (pole for carrying baskets) with taro and a bushel of bananas hanging from each side, indexing masculine plantation work. The scientist rhymes, "Vegetables and fruits, and that boy taro. You won't have any more sickness but emerging is the muscle," as the young man lifts the amo like a barbell. Another local fitness instructor posted a meme equating plantation labor with lifting weights. The photo shows two young men walking on the road with an amo supported by their shoulders. The caption says, "You lift? Nah we do *feaus* [chores]." The text links exercise assisted by gym equipment with the labor of plantation workers as these two young men carry coconut husks mounted to an amo, again linking a Samoan everyday planation technology with exercise equipment. Across health promotion materials, there is simultaneously blaming of culture, particularly in food values, and valorization of the physical fitness needed to be an active member of a family, caring for the land, and caring for the self.

Living in Samoa taught me that some differences really matter—rank, age, and gender all shaped how people treated each other in everyday life where equity was not expected. I came to accept these distinctions and the ways that they made resources flow (or not) as a taken-for-granted way of organizing the world. In a context where inequality is accepted, and conventionally exaggerated as a way of showing respect, talking about other forms of inequality—that is, inequality in life chances—was difficult. To talk about individual suffering, feeling cash strapped, or worrying about feeding one's family were statements that implicitly related to the failure of conventional systems of reciprocity to take care of every-one, even if in unequal ways. While people from a variety of religious backgrounds would critique the ways norms and practices around reciprocity were broken, Pentecostal Christianity in particular integrated a focus on how the global economy has brought about unequal life chances. In this way, while biomedical and public health efforts tended to reinforce a stereotype of local, and specifically Pacific, cultural factors that increased risk for disease, thus blaming "culture," Pentecostals refocused healing on the effort of *becoming* and the overwhelming pride that many have in the Christianity of Samoans (see Farmer 2003). Health identities, thrust upon people in the Pacific Islands, where obesity and diabetes rates are high, are stigmatized—foods deemed unappetizing by Euro-American standards are thought to be relished, as are large bodies. Pentecostalism, in contrast, provided a way to anchor identity in healing—striving to align self, body, and society in mutually beneficial ways, sustaining a spiritualized approach to living with cardiometabolic disorders, and addressing the ambiguities that arise from rapid change.

Food and fat are processes as much as materials. Becoming fat is a moral compass through which food and fitness gain their meaning. Thinking about materials like food and fat as processes is to say that they are created, and recreated, through mundane activities of cooking, talk, and prayer. Drawing from Janelle Taylor, food, fat, and fitness "materialize bodily surfaces" and provide ethnographers with "significant sites" for understanding broader social processes (2005, 742). In this case, food and fat were concepts that were ambiguous in the Samoan context because of rising economic inequalities where well-being generated from traditional means of resource sharing and redistribution was questioned as a means of unscrupulous accumulation. Looking to how the features of the body—like bellies, hunger, or physical movement—are created is a social process, which should encourage scholars and practitioners alike to stop associating fat positivity with cardiometabolic risk and instead refocus on developing locally meaningful measures of vulnerability. The macro trends presented above, followed by the ways that Samoan explanations for the emergence of these disorders sometimes contradict and sometimes support these trends, show one alignment—discerning risk is about discerning vulnerability in access to cash and supportive relationships. While public health and biomedicine in Samoa struggled to account for these kinds of experiences, Pentecostal Christianity, with its integration of biological and spiritual sources of suffering, helped born-again people articulate social risk as cardiometabolic risk. These examples present a cultural theory of social change as a generator of sickness, where *how* one gains weight matters in determining *if* one is sick or well.

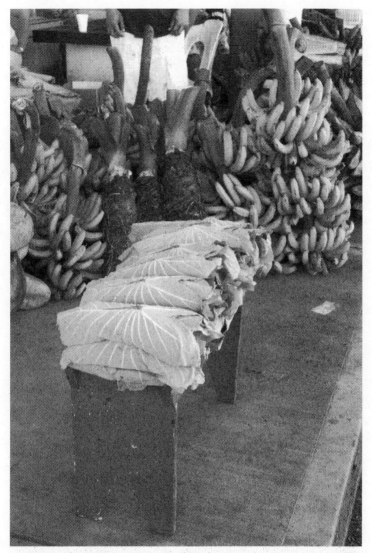

FIGURE 5 Buses chug along, taxis line up, and vendors sit fanning themselves as people wander through the market. Along the edges of the open-air market, vendors sell large starches like taro or ta'amu while the interior stalls focus on smaller, sometimes seasonal items like tomatoes, leafy greens, ripe bananas, cabbage, oranges, papaya, and cucumbers. Each vendor sells some combination of the same items, and each vendor prices the items similarly. The homogeneity of the offerings is remarkable. Those working in agriculture policy would often reflect on this, calling this trend the "cucumber mentality." It meant that farmers would see other vendors making money selling cucumbers, which would inspire them to grow cucumbers. Then shortly thereafter, everyone in the market starts growing cucumbers. They would describe this as flooding the market, which would drive down prices to the point where no vendor made any profit—the result: everyone abandons cucumber farming.

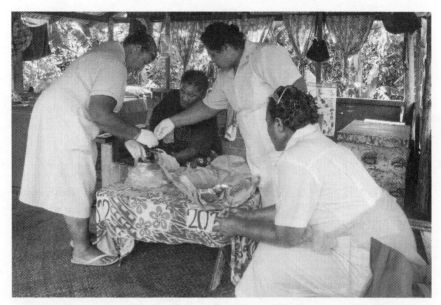

FIGURE 6 Being from *kua* (the back) is associated with old ways, sometime backwards ways. It suggested being uneducated, and poor. As we drove, the nurses explained we were going kua first, because these cases needed the most attention. On our first stop, the nurses bounded from their van to meet this man who was working in his plantation as we arrived. Without words, he acknowledged their arrival by walking to his fale. He lost his finger a few weeks earlier. He had cut himself with his machete while working in the plantation. He was also diabetic—he'd learn this when he went to the hospital. The finger had become infected and then necrotic, beyond recovery, so it was amputated. The nurses checked in on him every other day, changing the dressing each time. They brought a set of tools from the hospital, wrapped in paper, for each patient they visited. They left him with fresh bandages, and when possible, they would instruct someone else in the household on how to change the dressing. This man was alone, so they had no one to teach.

# 4 · FREEDOM AND HEALTH RESPONSIBILITY

McDonald's at 6:30 in the morning is quiet, dark, and cool from the air conditioning. I order an ice coffee, with no milk or sugar. The person behind the counter asks, "With nothing?" Yes, "no milk, no sugar, no flavor," I say. Minutes later, I am served a coffee with milk and gritty with sugar, like every other time I order coffee at McDonald's. Black coffee did not translate. Mele and I would sometimes meet at McDonald's before the clinic opened, and occasionally she would invite other staff and "shout" breakfast, paying for their hash browns, hotcakes, egg McMuffins, and milky, sugary coffees before the start of the morning shift at the clinic. When Mele returned to Samoa from living in New Zealand, she felt "so much had changed" and everything "cost money now, especially *meafai* [obligations]."[1] Mele and her husband returned to start a new Pentecostal church, and in recognizing how much life had changed in Samoa, she decided to work, even though the church would typically support the *faletua* (pastor's wife). Thus, her "shouting" at McDonald's was related to her mission as a faletua, to create a community where the congregants were not expected to provide for leaders, like the pastor, or superiors in the clinic; rather she would provide a "spiritual feed" or a "real feed" when needed—even if it was McDonald's, which she didn't see as a contradiction, given her work as a nurse.

This metaphor of feeding the congregation, or actually feeding her staff or families in her church, was integral to how Mele and her husband understood their own obligations to their community. Obligations refer to all the things—materials, time, cash—that families contribute to their extended families or church. Some obligations occur regularly—school fees and weekly alms, for example—while others need to be met on demand as family and church leaders make requests for special events, like fa'alavelave. Pentecostal churches actively reframed their obligations with the biblical metaphor of the shepherd tending to his sheep, to suggest that leaders should provide for their communities. This was different from the more typical model of Samoan leadership where communities provided for the leader and the leader gave back as needed. Pentecostal pastors and their families were differently obligated to congregations first, and congregants were obligated to God, not the pastor. As a result of this reframing, Mele felt her congregants chose her church because they felt "free," in contrast to their experiences with family where tautua and fa'aaloalo guided everyday interactions. This change is significant because it redirected responsibility for relationships from the community who served respected leaders to leaders who must serve their communities. One of the clearest ways to understand this Samoan notion of responsibility is through the proverb *o le ala i le pule o le* tautua ("the road to power is service"), which highlights the importance of serving based on role obligations determined by age, gender, kin, and/or title. The proverb articulates the moral obligation to serve community leaders through material forms like cash and food gifts or by giving one's labor, for example, by helping to build a church or working on the family plantation.

These social obligations ideologically define Samoan-ness—to serve is a way to be noticed by those in titled positions so to eventually secure one of those titles. Service, though, is more than a means to accumulating power; it also "glorifies" families. Everyday life in Samoa is beset with obligation where tautua and fa'aaloalo guide how one should interact in ways that create webs of obligations between people and groups and that instantiate expectations for action based on social roles. Role expectations determine how one should act and in turn how one should serve and therefore demonstrate respect for those older or ranked. The proverb mentioned above—"the road to power is service"—articulates the moral obligation to serve community leaders. Service and demonstrations of respect are thus a modus operandi for social interactions. In this context, freedom ideologies were novel in Samoa because they valorized individual action and motivation and thus countered Samoan notions of agency where "the dramatis personae rather than individuals" were thought to be the source of action (Duranti 1992, 27).[2] Christian notions of responsibility are markedly different. Typically, the Christian subject is positioned as a free subject—one who is free from obligations imposed by kin or culture (see Keane 2007). Responsibility is only possible when individuals are understood to be free, because for choice to be possible, or moral and sincere, one must live in a state of freedom from social obligation. Christianity necessarily depends on the freedom to choose salvation, and invoking freedom "acts as the guarantee of one's sincerity" (Keane 2007, 214).

Mele's invocation of freedom stood in direct contrast to the everyday realities of obligations, which presented daily contradictions around health choices. Just as Mele would advise her patients to avoid sugary tea and fatty foods yet would "shout" her staff breakfast at McDonald's, healthcare professionals often accepted food gifts of the very same foods they would advise patients to avoid. I spent a few weeks doing home visits with a group of nurses who traveled to remote parts of the main island to follow up with patients discharged from the hospital. Most of the patients we visited were suffering from complications from unmanaged diabetes, including wounds that would not heal. Most discussion was focused on "the worst" patients, those who refused to take their medications or continued to eat "all the bad foods" despite their knowledge, often with a recent diagnosis, that they had one or more cardiometabolic disorders. However, even as the nurses condemned patients, they welcomed meals of fried chicken and rice prepared by their families. In other instances, family members would chase down our van as we pulled away to slip a few cans of *pisupo* (tinned corned beef) through the windows, to "show their love for the work we do," the head nurse would explain. These mundane gifts and examples of feeding muddy the line between health and well-being, as patients and providers sometimes felt that individual health could often only be preserved at the expense of social well-being. They could only be respected as authoritative if they accepted these gifts, even while advising against them.

Across Samoa, refusing food or food gifts for health reasons—what would be considered a responsible thing to do to manage one's health—proved to be a "practical impossibility" for most people I encountered (Carr 2015, 281). When Mele fed her staff McDonald's, or the nurses accepted gifts of tinned meats, they felt they were caring for the social relationships that structured their working lives, even if this meant eating or gifting foods that were otherwise considered off limits for those living with cardiometabolic disorders. In addition to the health dilemmas posed by eating and feeding, providing foods that were good for relationships was increasingly costly. As I spent time with Pentecostal people, I found that the language of freedom provided a vocabulary for reflecting on these impracticalities. By this, I mean Pentecostals learned to see themselves before they were born again as "unfree," that is, constrained by family, tradition, and egotistical concerns with status and pride. With conversion, they identified a new prioritization of their individual relationship with God as creating the experience of freedom—a newfound pleasure and sense of urgency in focusing attention on one's relationship with God through prayer, fasting, and Bible study. When narrating illness experiences, freedom provided a vocabulary to link the experiences of stress, depression, anger, and other negative emotions with social constraints. This vocabulary introduced a Christian framework for reflecting on the limitations of individual agency, while simultaneously valorizing efforts toward cultivating individual agency. In other words, when Pentecostals used the language of freedom, they pointed to how they wanted to be healthier, but their family lives made that nearly impossible.

Newfound experiences of freedom helped to explain new positive impacts of opting out of obligations—healing, feeling at peace. While it may seem that freedom bolstered the individual as independent, instead freedom provided a Christian framework for understanding the self in relation to God and indirectly to others. Freedom was a state of striving to develop one's faith. In talking about freedom and sickness together, the striving dimensions of Christian personhood were extended to health. By narrating how freedom was an ideal state, those living with or supporting others with cardiometabolic disorders attuned to determining who was responsible for health and illness. To say someone was "unfree" was to implicitly point to the social constraints that made that person sick. Freedom discourses, thus, expressed a particular set of ideas about social responsibility—the individual should be unburdened by social expectations to have a true and authentic relationship with God—and formed a Pentecostal analytic for understanding sociality. To be free was to reflect on one's place in the world and to evaluate one's obligations to God, family, and church. In this context, well-being was defined by the freedom to choose how to fulfill social obligations while health was the result of experiencing what it meant to be free.

This convergence of freedom discourses and ideas about health shows how etiologies are political; they are religious theories about the "uneven distribution of life chances" (Carney 2015a, 164). Like other ethnographers, I am interested in how etiologies are more than "'local' or 'cultural' (subjective) understandings of illness" that require "my own analytical lens to describe the 'real' or 'factual' (objective) ways in which power inequalities produce and distribute illness" (Hamdy 2008, 553). Instead, I focus on how my interlocutors "make both of these analytical moves when they make meaning out of illness" (Hamdy 2008, 553). Freedom ideologies helped my interlocutors make both of these "analytical moves" by clarifying how obligations, which were increasingly difficult to meet, were sources of suffering. Freedom ideologies collapsed the distinction between "what is a health problem and what is a social problem," creating a Pentecostal framework of social suffering (Kleinman 2010, 1519). Scholarly attention to social suffering explores how diseases caused by socioeconomic inequalities create suffering that is not only individual, but extends into the family or other social networks (Kleinman, Das, and Lock 1997). For Pentecostal Samoans, social suffering was defined by the experiences of stress, anger, and depression generated from obligation, which by extension were thought to cause cardiometabolic disorders. According to this etiology, emotional suffering generated physical sickness, creating metabolic imbalance in ways that only spiritual healing could ameliorate. Healing depended on restoring spiritual balance.

When freedom discourses were mobilized to understand health and sickness, they challenged biomedical discourses that tended to naturalize the responsibilization of individual citizens (Berlant 2007; LeBesco 2011; Trnka 2017). Responsibilization refers to the neoliberal process of shifting responsibility from the state, or other institutions, to the individual. This reflects a neoliberal form of agency, where "people own themselves as though they were a business" (Gershon 2011, 539). In turn, "the problems of problematic persons are reformulated as moral or ethical problems" (Rose 2000, 334). With this transfer of responsibility comes new expectations for citizens to self-cultivate attention. When applied to cardiometabolic disorders, this makes self-care (in the form of regular blood glucose testing or weight management) a moral duty (Berlant 2007, 757). Glucometers and scales, in this way, are freedom "technologies" that publicly demonstrate individual responsibility (see also Rose 1999). Assigning responsibility is thus a way to know the body and make certain kinds of relationships with others. However, these neoliberal notions of the responsible citizen are not "watertight" (Trnka and Trundle 2014, 141). In everyday life, responsibility is more complex, especially when viewed in relation to care relations, where action is motivated by the well-being of others (Trnka and Trundle 2014, 136). This notion of care has a long heritage in Christian thought, where Christians have an "obligation to promote the well-being of the wider community and extend compassion toward the vulnerable" (Trnka and Trundle 2014, 136, 2017; Elisha 2011). When Pentecostals used freedom discourses to talk about illness, they articulated what health scholars have suggested for many years, that cardiometabolic disorders are not the fault of the individual but rather the result of complex social, economic, and ecological interactions. The trope of freedom shows a retooling of social responsibility, where Pentecostals reflected on the impossibilities of embracing individualized health responsibility within a context of gifting, eating, and feeding. The ways Pentecostals used the language of freedom shows that those living with cardiometabolic disorders did not wholesale integrate the notion of individual health responsibility as communicated through biomedicine and public health. Instead, they strove toward individualized responsibility through their relationship with God and, in turn, reflected on the myriad factors that contributed to their health or sickness.

## THE STRESS OF OBLIGATION, THE PEACE OF FREEDOM

> For us; family…family unity…name…reputation…appearances…
> privacy…are EVERYTHING. It's almost sacrilegious to prioritize the
> individual, the "needs of the one," over "the needs of the many." It can be
> seen as the epitome of selfishness.
>
> —Lani Wendt Young (2013)

A lawyer in his midforties, Sione was born again minutes before entering the hospital for preparatory dialysis surgery.[3] When he reflected on why he was born again, he used the language of freedom, saying, "We shuffle in and you sit down and you stand up for hymns and you sit down and there's no interactive worship." More importantly, "there's no expectation that there's any other response from the congregation other than maybe reading the Bible out loud. It's not like in the new churches where you are free to express yourself." Sione's words articulated the dissatisfaction some experienced in their mainline churches, namely obligation to perform. "That's your time, just singing the hymns," he said. When I asked why he attended his family church despite feeling dissatisfied, he responded, "Because of the *fa'asāmoa*." In other words, he continued to go to church because it was essential to being a good son, husband, and brother. He knew that he was there for this reason, because of obligations, not because he could experience God—reflecting the comments above by Lani Wendt Young, a prominent Samoan author. Referencing fa'asāmoa was a way to reiterate the idea that family and reputation should guide decision making, not desire for an individually satisfying experience of church.

I had heard about Sione's "miraculous" recovery as stories of his healing circulated widely at Glory House. He was skeptical, at first, about Pentecostal churches, but when he learned that he needed surgery, he attended a healing service in New Zealand. This was the first time Sione had "felt anything" in church, and he contrasted this with feeling "empty" at his family church. He could "feel the power" during the healing service because he knew that "people all around the world [were] praying" for him. This last point was particularly important to Sione; he felt his own church was not praying for him, while people he didn't even know in Pentecostal churches "around the world" were praying for him. This knowledge of the work of a prayer warrior network revealed the problem of obligation to Sione.[4] His church made demands of him, but when it came time for him, the church "just depended on the doctors." It seemed to him that even strangers cared more about him than his own family and church.

At the healing service, Sione approached the pastor about "receiving healing." When he told the pastor about his kidney disease, the pastor laid hands on his shoulders, instructing him to "breathe out, breathe it all out." When Sione took a deep breath, he "felt something, something warm and hot." He felt as if he was being "immersed in a warm oil bath." Then he knew the disease "came out, not just [his] breathe, but other things come out too." He felt this "symbolized" his kidney disease leaving his body, which he came to see as a *ma'i ona o le faiga o mea 'uma* ("sickness of doing all the things"), a sickness derived from the stress of meeting expectations. He had so much "stress before," generated from feeling the need to fulfill weekly cash contributions to his family. He felt this stress acutely even though, as a lawyer, he earned a comparatively handsome salary. However, once he started attending his Pentecostal church, Sione felt he had "the freedom to express [his] joy," and as a result, he was "happier and healthier" because his "heart was healed."

When Sione described feeling freedom, he critiqued how his obligations once dominated how he related to God. Often, when I would ask people about their health, they would respond with reflections on their obligations. Sitting in the outdoor corridors between hospital wards, Losa, a widowed prayer warrior in her early fifties, whispered, as she thumbed through the tattered pages of her Bible, "I did a lot for the church. The fundraising and obligations for the church." Losa felt pressed for money all the time, making it clear to her that she didn't give "out of faith, free will." Instead, she felt "forced." The pastor encouraged her family to give "the maximum amount" and she felt she was giving all the time: "You con-

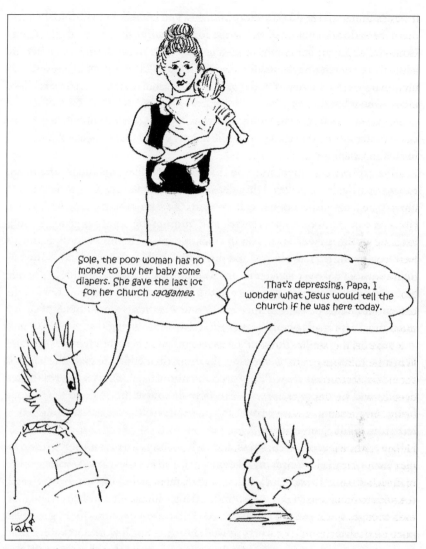

FIGURE 7 This regularly appearing cartoon takes controversial issues and narrates them from the perspective of a father, "Papa," and his son, "Sole." They are playful, cued by the fact that sole is an informal way that young men refer to each other, something akin to "brother." Cartoon from the *Samoa Observer*, January 2, 2012.

tribute a thousand for this, a hundred for this, you know?" But what, I asked, did this have to do with her diabetes? These constant contributions made her family "struggle," she said; her family "tried and tried hard to earn money to meet the need of the church." Shyly, she told me her family was very poor as a result, saying, "In my family, there was nothing." This contrasted to her experience at Glory House where "we do everything with our free will." The "stress" of constant searching for resources to give to family churches, she felt, also eventually led to the death of her husband because of complications due to diabetes, which I explore further in Chapter Five.

Losa expressed a common trope that I heard in many iterations. The newspaper, in particular, articulated this idea with some regularity: "Our willingness to give is a beautiful aspect of our culture" and "there is nothing wrong with giving when we can." However, Lesa also felt that "most of the time, our giving is motivated by wrong reasons," like "fear of embarrassment." In other words, Samoans were not "giving from the heart," and this was a "problem" (Lesa 2012b). The cartoon above articulates this skepticism in a drawing of a mother unable to provide basic needs for her children because of the demands of church obligations. Sole, the son, responds to Papa, grimly wondering what Jesus would think of such a situation. These kinds of critiques suggest that while giving is supposed to provide support for families through the development of generous networks of families, instead people were made vulnerable from their efforts to give. The paradox persists, and critiques are widely shared and normalized, even while extoling the benefits and virtues of reciprocity. Freedom discourses normalized the critique further by focusing on the spiritual and physical results of social suffering generated from fulfilling obligations.

The relationship of illness, stress, and cash poverty also became real to me over the course of my fieldwork as my relationship with Telisa developed. Telisa worked in Apia, had earned a bachelor's degree in the United States, and acted as a research consultant for me, answering questions, working with me on translations and transcriptions, and as a general confidant. As Telisa and I became closer, she began asking for advances for her work, or would rush to finish work some weeks and then work more slowly in other weeks. Later, I realized that this pace reflected the changing needs of her family. In weeks when obligations were high, Telisa would work furiously. During other weeks, she would take her time because she did not need additional cash and to have cash made her vulnerable to giving it away. Despite Telisa's full-time employment in a desirable position, she was still always in need of cash. Speedy work, going to work without lunch, and talking about only eating taro for dinner were all shorthand ways to talk about struggling with cash.

One reason why Telisa had so many obligations was that her house was built on freehold land, which attracted youth from her natal village who wanted to go to school in Apia or just wanted to get away from their own rural households.

When I met Telisa, there were seven people living in her house; within a year, there were twelve people. As the only employed person, Telisa was responsible for the everyday needs of the family, including food, sundries, school fees, utilities, family debts for the house and the car, and, finally, for fa'alavelave, which her mother determined. Telisa felt she was inextricably tied to webs of reciprocity but was not receiving any support. This led to resentment that fulfilling these obligations was at the expense of fulfilling her own plans, as she dreamed of building her own home on her own land.

Telisa converted while I worked with her, in search of "freedom," she said. Shortly thereafter, she realized that, "Church didn't have to be so stressful. Church should be a place for peace." Once Telisa started worshipping on Sundays at a Pentecostal church, and stopped attending her family's church, she began to feel free, she told me. She also explained that she thought her gout (a weight-related chronic condition) was caused by the stress of trying to provide for her family. She even felt that since her conversion, she hadn't had the same foot pain associated with gout, and as a result, she was walking in the evenings for exercise, which she felt helped her lose weight.

When Pentecostals cited freedom as a major reason for being born again, it allowed them to take on a position of making a choice to support one's family—an agentive stance. Freedom discourses helped people use cardiometabolic disorders as embodied metaphors for talking about the burdens of obligation where a lack of choice caused sickness. Freedom, therefore, articulated the ability to make choices in how one supported family. The language helped people to create a stance toward responsibility to God first, then family. It created a conceptual space to choose health, even if that choice was sometimes inconsequential to changing health metrics. Sione began to see the stress of meeting family expectations as the source of his kidney disease; Losa saw her husband's constant searching for money to meet obligations as the source of the complications that eventually led to his death; Telisa felt the stress of meeting church demands caused her gout and made it difficult for her to prevent flare-ups. Freedom discourses brought into focus anxieties about the endemic hierarchies that each of these people managed every day by focusing on the effects this had on the body. By focusing on the embodied effects of obligation, Pentecostals critiqued values that guided everyday Samoan life—respect, generosity, and hierarchical obedience—in ways that valorized their Christian identities as free.

## THE LIMITS OF CHOICE

One afternoon I sat with Ilo, a pastor, in his air-conditioned office at Glory House to see if he knew anyone healed from *suka* or *toto*. "They are healed, I'm 100% sure we are healed," he said. "When we pray, we are healed. But the trouble is they go back to sinful ways." From Ilo's perspective, healing was always complete, but individuals were responsible for bringing it into being through faith, and for managing their suka or toto. If faith dwindled, or as Ilo would describe, if people were to "lose sight of God," their health might suffer. The completeness of healing was subjunctive—healing could be complete if faith persisted (see also Bialecki 2017). He offered himself as an example, saying, "I was delivered from the spirit of suka and toto, but it's me." He advised people who sought healing from him, "I always tell people when you pray, you can heal. But it does not mean you go back and eat the same food. But I never question the healing." Ilo never questioned the effectiveness of God's healing, but he did talk about how his diet was largely out of his control because of the cost of food. "The trouble is, tomorrow, I eat the same food," he said. He wished he could change it, but instead he was praying for more money to "buy all these vegetables," which he hoped would allow his healing to be complete. While Ilo felt he was healed, he realized his health did not always change because of his own actions—he would smile as he told me he really enjoyed eating pork and lu'au (baby taro leaves cooked in coconut cream). The perfectness of healing showed Ilo that something else was keeping him sick, the cost of food perhaps, which was out of his control. Making different choices was impractical and sometimes impossible.

For others, the limits of choice for one generation could be inherited through the generations, explaining familial patterns of cardiometabolic disorders. Elia, a prayer intercessor at Glory House, was born again when she visited her father in New Zealand, where he had just suffered a stroke and was dying. When Elia visited him in the hospital, she began to feel that his sickness was not something the hospital doctors could heal and began to wonder about spiritual causes. Her sister agreed, saying, "That's just the way he is"—his anger and depression made him sick. They arranged to have a Pentecostal pastor visit their father, so "he could be saved," which would "make him free." Elia's father listened to the pastor, he cried, and Elia felt for the first time that "the Holy Spirit opened [his] heart." At this moment, Elia also had a vision of her grandfather hitting her father, and explained to me that "my grandfather drank too much, and they didn't have anything"—they were cash poor. Realizing that her grandfather's problems were caused by the "spirit of addiction," creating poverty in their family, helped her to understand why her own father was so angry and depressed. The family members who stood by their father's bedside were each born again and "prayed for forgiveness" for the entire family to stop the inheritance of depression and anger between generations. This multigenerational anger and depression explained, she said, "why [her] father was sick."

More concretely, some interlocutors addressed the costs of healthy foods through prayer, which helped them make different choices. Masina, a woman in her forties who was an AOG church member, told me she had suka and toto because she couldn't change her diet. She went to the doctor because she had an enduring headache, was diagnosed with suka and toto, and was advised to avoid "salty foods and the fats." Masina worked in Apia and she struggled with changing her diet for three reasons. First, she needed to eat while at work, and so she purchased foods that were mostly "the bad ones," because they were the only affordable options that did not require preparation—instant noodles, pork buns, and potato chips. Second, most people working in offices do not bring their own lunch, so to bring one's own lunch is to choose to eat alone. One friend told me she was trying to get her husband to eat healthier, so she started preparing his lunch. Surprisingly, her husband began to gain weight, and when she asked him about it, he said he would eat his prepared lunch on the bus and then go out to eat with his work colleagues for lunch as he didn't want to seem like he was avoiding their company. Finally, and more specific to Masina and her husband, they had small children and no other adults living with them. Therefore, there was no one available to grow food, and they had no land because they lived in an urban area. As a result, Masina purchased most of their foods, which meant "changing [her] mentality" about what she bought—she had to spend more than she wanted on foods that were "healthy." She prayed for the strength to make different choices when she went to the markets, which helped her "spend more on things like vegetables and more expensive [lean] meat." She also began to "pray for the food to bring God's healing," as she felt her healing came from "God's strength to keep the diet." Masina used prayer as a resource to make changes in her life, which allowed her to make budgeting choices in a way that was morally satisfying; she was obeying God's demands to "treat [her] body as the temple God created." Choosing to spend money on lean meats, fruits, and vegetables necessarily meant contributing less to her extended family, even though the demands continued.

Pentecostal health practitioners also had particularly clear explanations for the rise of cardiometabolic disorders that focused on how relationships often limited choice. One afternoon, I talked with Mareta, a Tongan physician I interviewed ten times over two years, at her favorite coffee shop. Mareta thought her rapid weight gain and health problems started when she was one of the only Tongan women at university in Fiji, because she felt isolated and depressed. Her Samoan boyfriend and future husband insisted that she visit his Pentecostal church to help her feel better. After the first service, Mareta said she "loved the free feeling, like [she] could just do what [she] felt." She said, "I didn't have to worry who knew me, or who knew I was Tongan, or even [who knew] my family."

Despite feeling like she had found a "church home," Mareta still struggled with loneliness. As she continued her medical studies, she felt her "knowledge of how the Holy Spirit works" continue to grow, and so she developed parallel explanations for why cardiometabolic disorders were on the rise across Samoa and in her own life. "The medical literature," she said, shows that there are "so many disorders or diseases where stress plays a big part." Stress was derived from "spiritual roots" like "bitterness" and "fear," which caused cardiometabolic sickness. These spirits "disturb the normal balance of things, chemicals and hormones in the body, and therefore you lose your health and this leads to diseases." In her case, her isolation caused stress and depression, which introduced evil spirits into her body, which had a cardiometabolic effect on the body—creating high levels of suka and toto.

"For me," she explained, "I've always had this thing of self-hate." Her weight was a daily reminder of that feeling, which only increased after she graduated from university because, during her medical training, she learned that her weight should be under individual control, and yet she still didn't feel she had the "strength to change, even though [she] knew better." In other words, she neither changed her diet nor exercised because her suffering from feeling isolated endured. Mareta had the added stress of feeling like her relationship with her husband was always under attack because she was a Tongan woman married to a Samoan man, living in Samoa. "Women don't treat our marriage as real," she said. Additionally, her husband was a "big fitness guy" and "very handsome." He was supportive of her health, when he hiked up the small mountain in the urban area—a popular place for urban residents to engage in physical activity—he invited her. He also cooked dinners rich with vegetables. However, she felt this "support" was added pressure to lose weight, further deepening her feelings of "self-hate." Mareta was, therefore, struggling again, as she did in university, with loneliness and isolation. Crying during our meetings, Mareta felt guilty because she had "the knowledge of medicine," and believed that if she just dieted and exercised, she would lose weight and control her suka. Yet, she did not seem able to change her eating, nor could she bring herself to exercise, so she turned to prayer to help heal these spirits of depression and stress, which she felt was the ultimate source of her fatness and sickness.

Tavī, a physician in her late forties, also articulated the ways that relationships might limit choice. Tavī opened a clinic with a Christian mission—to heal the whole person, "mind, body, and spirit." Citing the Gospel of Mark, Tavī explained, "Even in the Bible there are doctors. Jesus said, 'Those who are well do not need a doctor, but those who are sick,' they do. Jesus came for the sinners and the sick. We are here to help them." Believing humans were made of three parts, she said, "We live in this body and we have a soul or emotions that control us." Human suffering, including sickness, she felt could be healed by addressing the "inner man," because this inner spirit "communes with the spirit of God." Tavī thought healing occurred in the body as a result of how she addressed the spirit in her clinic. Iterating a common Christian contrast between spirit and flesh, she felt most people "don't know" that "the flesh breeds corruption" and leads the body to die "piece by piece"—especially among those living with diabetes who face amputations "toe by toe." Food, in particular, was a tremendous source of "temptation," because "the flesh always leads you into things that bring trouble and strife. Sickness. Ill health." Good foods were especially dangerous.

Stress, as the cause of cardiometabolic disorders, resulted from being led by the flesh—by the desire to eat but also the desire to be noticed or to be seen as the strongest. Using appetite to talk about food and power, she explained, "Stress happens when we don't cast our burdens over to the Lord." This was particularly true for those living with cardiometabolic disorders, as "a big problem with suka and toto is the stress, worry, anxiety." When stress, worry, and anxiety rise, so do suka and toto, so she encouraged her patients to "cast your cares on the Lord for he cares for you." Sympathizing, she said "often we just take it back upon ourselves" instead of praying, so "we continue to worry about it." Tavī based her practice around the idea that stress resulted from being led by desire, or from the isolation of not seeking help, and this in turn created sickness. Healing created cardiometabolic balance as a reflection of an individual's connection to the "the spirit of God," so resulting in "spiritual balance."

These cases provide a diverse set of explanations for why cardiometabolic disorders endure. In each case, choice was limited, and freedom discourses provided a language for talking about these limitations. Scholarship in health research, often, has focused on the limitations that result from the high costs of imported foods and the lagging agricultural markets in Oceania. The narratives above, from Masina and Ilo, highlight the cost of food as prohibitive. However, participants also focused on other kinds of limitations that create suffering and that generate sickness. Mareta's recalcitrant fat was a reminder of her spiritual struggles. Tavī felt that distance from God had resulted in cardiometabolic imbalance. Elia believed anger and depression could be inherited in ways that caused high blood pressure resulting in a stroke. All used the language of freedom to articulate how social context limited individual abilities to create health. Responsibility rested with the individual for their health, *only if* the individual was free from the constraints of family and church. These examples also highlight the practical difficulties associated with eating, feeding, and gifting. These included relational responsibilities that impacted health, but also broader struggles—emotional suffering caused from relationships, stress, depression, and addiction—all of which created spiritual and cardiometabolic imbalances. Freedom signaled a perspective where one was opting to first and foremost relate to God, thus authorizing people to place conventional obligations as secondary. This stance had micro consequences for daily eating, feeding, and gifting habits, as well as macro consequences shaping what it meant to be a responsible family or community member. Living with and managing cardiometabolic disorders thus involved more than shifting diet and exercise behaviors; it required shifting the locus of how one related to others.

## PRACTICING FREEDOM

Freedom discourses encouraged reflection on responsibilities to self, community, and God—something Mele's church was actively developing to help congregants identify constraints as a way of striving toward individual responsibility. A fifteen-minute drive from Apia along a dirt road, Mele's church was a simple concrete building, painted white with no sign indicating the purpose of the building. While some congregations prided themselves on the beauty of their church buildings, sometimes spending millions of *tālā* to build new structures, Mele's church was ordinary by design. The structure was indicative of how Mele and her husband aimed to cultivate freedom—its simplicity reflected the minimal material obligations of the congregants to church. Their obligations were to God. At McDonald's, Mele told me about what it was like when they first opened the church. The children were sick, "weak and filthy." Infected scabies and the dirty noses of church children, she felt, were evidence of parental neglect that ultimately indicated that the families were "unfree." The parents were "stressed all the time, running around trying to find money and leaving the children to themselves." She felt that being consumed with obligation, in a context where there was little opportunity to earn cash, made her "congregants desperate and sick," like so many of her diabetes clinic patients as well. By being free, Mele felt, Pentecostals could create intimacy with God because they were unburdened by the obligations of kin and church. For Mele, freedom expressed a particular set of ideas about social responsibility—the individual should be unburdened by social expectations to have a true relationship with God—and articulates a Pentecostal analytic for understanding sociality. To be free was to reflect on reciprocity and the multiple obligations that come with participation in family and community life—not to abstain *per se*. In this context, well-being was defined by the freedom to *choose* how to fulfill social obligations, while health was the result of experiencing what it meant to be free. Mele and her husband explicitly cultivated freedom through three primary measures: minimizing offerings and gifts, informality with congregants and especially youth, and gendered mentoring.

Mele did a number of things to reduce the obligation to give. First, she worked; as noted above, this was very uncommon for faletua across denominations. She found her work was her specific godly "mission," and she also explicitly wanted to lessen the burden on others to provide for the pastor's family. On a more symbolic level, Mele and her husband changed the Sunday service so they would not collect the offering during the service. As people entered the building, they could drop their money into a box located in front of the church. Most churches dedicated a section of the service to the offering, either circulating collection plates or by having families come to the front of the church to deposit their offerings, often accompanied by a prayer and song over the money. They also did not require congregants to decorate the church—it was common for church families to rotate this responsibility, with families often competing to provide the most extravagant flowers and fabrics to drape over the altar. Another symbolically important way that Mele and her husband aimed to reduce obligations was to prepare their own *to'ona'i* (Sunday lunch), which congregants typically prepared for the pastor's family either by delivering individual plates or rotating the responsibility among families. For example, when I lived with a pastor and his family, each night, congregants would deliver trays of food—soup, rice, fried chicken, taro, mutton flaps—enough to feed the large household of ten or more. In contrast, Mele and her family would eat their Sunday lunch at church, not retreating to their home, and they brought their own food. They aimed to create transparency: they showed congregants not only that they prepared their own foods, but also that they ate purposely simple and "healthy" foods, like fish and taro. They invited congregants to join—reinforcing Mele's pastoral idea that they should provide real food in addition to spiritual food when needed.

In these ways, Mele and her husband minimized public forms of competitive giving—that is, they created conventions that reduced public displays of giving in ways that made congregants feel less pressure to give. By reducing the obligation to give, Mele felt her congregants had greater economic well-being, which she could see since the church opened. Using church children again as an example, she explained, "They have, the kids, now they wear nice shoes. They walk in and they have their little dresses and clothes. They walk in and can feel good." Mele believed that if parents could direct their resources into family needs, including clothing, for example, over public demonstrations of wealth, like gifts of tinned beef and rice to the pastor and his family, they would be happier and healthier. Mele, therefore, communicated the meaning of freedom in economic terms, as the autonomy to direct resources to the nuclear family.

Mele also aimed to create intimacy with her congregants, especially youth, as a way of creating freedom. She told me about a conversation she had with a young girl and boy from her church to help me understand how intimacy and freedom were linked. "The normal ways we used to be," she said, was how she liked to be with her congregation. This imagined past suggested that the negative impact of obligations (where church was a space of competition) was new. She said, "Sometimes the girls, they say 'hey mama,'" marking an uncommon informality between church children and the faletua. A more typical image of a faletua was an old woman sitting in the front of the church using a long stick, perhaps four or five feet long, to tap the heads of misbehaving children sitting together under her watchful eye. Mele was purposely different, evidenced by the fact that a young girl would address her as "mama."

The young girl, Mele recounted, complained about the boy, saying, "I'm not happy with the way he talks to me, the way he looks at me." With expressive cheekiness, Mele says, "Who? Him! Why are you looking at her?" directing her gaze and widening her eyes to an imagined boy. Her church did not permit dating relationships among youth, she explained, raising an eyebrow, saying, "as they do in other churches." When Mele said, "in other churches," she drew attention to the disconnect between the formality of respect protocols and the enforcement of Christian rules. In conventional churches, as with Mele's church, youth were not permitted to date. However, in practice, youth did date and conduct romantic relationships. She thought that as long as youth played their role, serving and respecting elders, then the pastor and his family would ignore romantic indiscretions. Mele felt that her church was different because the youth could come to the pastor and the faletua about their relationships. Formality in the mainline churches, she suggested, made intimacy with congregants impossible, because congregants were too concerned with how they appeared in church. Freedom contrasted this formality, as it suggested choice and relief from the respect protocols that often guided the interactions of parents and children, pastors and congregants, and elders and youth. By cultivating intimacy with congregants and by decreasing formality, Mele and her husband sought to reduce congregants' concerns with how they appeared to church leaders, which she hoped would reduce how much money and time they felt compelled to commit to church.

Finally, Mele felt that the stress of obligation impacted relationships, particularly between husbands and wives. As with her assessment of the church children, Mele gauged the "spiritual health" of the church by looking to the "mothers of the church." She would say to them, "You need to look after yourself. I see you're still young. Some of you are much younger than me, but you look older. Why? Because you let yourself go. Why did you let yourself go?" They would say, "Oh, because I have children, and so many obligations." Mele felt the women were "letting themselves go" because they were stressed, prioritizing the needs of the extended family over caring for themselves and their husbands. Appearances—the cleanliness of clothes, hair styling, adornment—indexed well-being. Without attention to appearance, Mele worried that church mothers were putting their marriages in peril, and she reminded the women that their husbands "go out to work" and "look at other ladies" only to come home to find their wives at home "with no bra" wearing "the same shirt as they slept in the night before." She beseeched them, "What happened to the lady he married—the woman he fell in love with? Where's that girl?"

Mele argued that women neglected their appearances because of "the stress of all these obligations." By extension, Mele taught families how health and wealth were interconnected, where health was first linked to looking well, including by a tidy and clean appearance, not unlike the women's associations. She connected appearance to social care, again asking women, "Do you still love your husband? Then look after yourself. Make yourself look good. Do your hair." Sometimes she would even volunteer to come to their houses to style their hair. Gesturing to her hair, she said, "I put a little gel here, a little gel there. I wear earrings," to which the women in her church would laugh. By not looking after their appearances, Mele suggested that the women were not looking after their husbands and children. Equating care for the self with care for the family, Mele encouraged the women to spend resources, including time, labor, and cash, on their appearance as a way to show affection to their husbands. Intimacy with God, Mele felt, hinged on intimacy between family members, which required directing resources to the nuclear family and God over the extended family. She made this apparent when she said, "You need to show them, to remember that all these days are the days that have been given to you. So live your life free because one day you will be dead and you'll go upstairs [she pointed upward], not fa'alavelave and these things." In other words, to be free of obligation was to be responsible to God. Obligations "bound families," Mele said, referencing how evil spirits "bind" or trap people, making them "unfree." This made their "health bad, from the stress."

Mele's practices created the experience of freedom in multiple ways. First, these practices de-emphasized public evaluations of families, thereby reducing obligations to give to the church and the pastor and his family. By linking economic freedom with spiritual freedom, Mele's practices suggested that without economic obligation, congregants could be free of other forms of obligation, such as performing respect. In this way, economic autonomy was made equivalent to freedom from social assessment as a foundation from which individuals could then develop intimacy with God. Second, by creating informality, congregants could develop charismatic practice without being concerned with the watchful eye of church elders, which ultimately strengthened their relationship with God. Finally, Mele mentored women in the church to link stress from obligation with family well-being, encouraging them to direct resources to the self as a way of caring for nuclear family relationships. In Mele's wide category of well-being, financial choice was tied to prosperity in body and family. Freedom was the capacity to exercise autonomy.

## THE LIMITATIONS OF FREEDOM

Attention to freedom discourses—when they articulate as a critique of obligation or when they provide people with a reflexive stance from which to evaluate responsibility—shows how social causes of suffering are incorporated into key etiologies of cardiometabolic disorders. Freedom discourses generated discussions among congregants about responsibility in a variety of ways: freedom was associated with the choice to give and the ability to practice charismatically, to feel unconstrained by social expectations, and to turn to God for support. By using the language of freedom, Pentecostals created a critical stance toward obligation, allowing them to carefully examine the social links that they created through their reciprocity with others. While the anthropology of Christianity has thoroughly explored how Christian practice ideologically focuses on individual salvation and sincerity, bringing medical anthropological perspectives to the topic of freedom reveals how healing generates commentary on the relationship between individual and community well-being. These freedom discourses challenge everyday hierarchies and deep expectations that one should act according to one's role, which are increasingly difficult to sustain in the current context of rising inequalities. Pentecostal freedom discourses drew attention to the limitations of choice by linking spiritual suffering, economic hardship, and distance from God with sickness. In this way, freedom discourses are social tools for talking about the shifting quality of responsibility. Sometimes, responsibility was a choice, as in fulfilling one's obligations to God, and other times, responsibility was compelled by families, as in fa'alavelave obligations. Pentecostal churches did not forbid kin-based reciprocity, but they did want congregants to choose to fulfill their obligations, not doing so automatically or for the wrong reasons. Freedom discourses clarified these differences. Sometimes, individuals needed to change their eating habits, which they could only do with the assistance of prayer; other times, people needed to redirect resources from extended family to nuclear family. In still other cases, relationships needed healing as a way of changing health. Freedom discourses encouraged reflection upon responsibility and obligation, but ultimately this did little to challenge the inequalities that could make eating, feeding, and gifting so challenging.

When Pentecostals used the language of freedom, they saw themselves as having a choice in how they engaged with their church and family. However, these ideologies did not always change how they engaged their church and family, nor could they always withdraw from difficult relationships. Freedom discourses challenged some obligations that shaped the experience of social suffering, but did not entirely transform them. They highlighted the experience of economic hardship but neglected the encompassing structural shifts that created an environment in the islands where cash was required for social reproduction, and yet opportunities to earn were limited. Using the language of freedom clarified how people were constrained by social relations, but not the political economy.

Despite this, these religious discourses were central to how Pentecostals made the experiences of cardiometabolic disorders meaningful. While it would seem on the surface that freedom discourses would entrench notions of individual responsibility, the vocabulary helped people to translate how pressures related to macro trends of urbanization and changes in global food trade impacted individuals and families through cash poverty, stress, addiction, and depression. Pentecostals therefore articulated the social origins of illness through an experiential focus on personal stress, generated by perceived lack of control of resources. This focus on the connection between stress and cardiometabolic disorders shows how healing is not only about changing orientations to the body, but also about changing orientations to relationships. Freedom discourses, as some of these cases show, can influence health practices—encouraging people to take medication, modify food intake, or increase physical activity, as well reduce alcohol and smoking. When people talked about the freedom that came with conversion, they felt they had a choice—to make health a priority—despite very real limitations. In fact, freedom discourses encouraged people to talk about those limitations as a means to change those challenges using their faith as the primary means of transformation.

Pentecostalism, however, did not change the material conditions of people's lives in all cases. Some of my interlocutors admitted to giving more of their resources to the church with conversion, but their orientation to responsibility changed. Many came to experience "joy" because of their intimacy with God. They came to aspire to closeness with God in ways that created a sense of well-being, despite struggles to maintain health and despite that their social and economic circumstances may not have changed. Pentecostals felt that they were responsible for their faith, and, in turn, if stress continued, or fat persisted, they remembered to turn to God to change their health behaviors. The transformative potential of healing thus lay in religious, not individual, change.

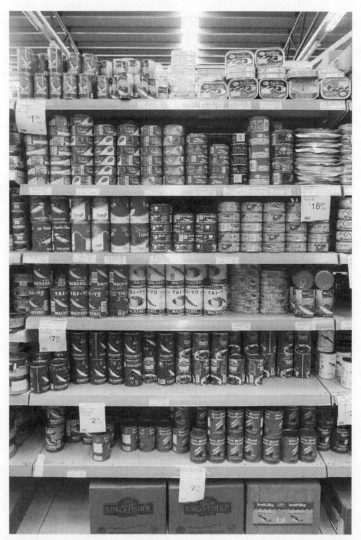

FIGURE 8 The tinned fish aisle is my favorite aisle in the supermarket because it is so colorful and tidy. A whole aisle is dedicated to stacked cans of fish and corned beef, so full that cases of cans are stored on the floor underneath the shelves. Tuna was expensive, but if you were lucky you had family in American Samoa who would bring cans of wahoo, which were not available in Samoa. Mackerel was the preferred tinned fish, but sardines with tomato sauce would do when budgets were especially tight. In sandwiches with mayonnaise or mixed with rice or noodles, the soft fish was often crunchy, as the little bones of the fish remained. Whenever visiting someone, I would bring a plastic bag of tinned items, a little pisūpo (always the best brand, Palm), tuna, and mayonnaise. In my early days of fieldwork, I'd bring baskets of vegetables, but I soon learned that these store-bought items were recognized as gifts, while the vegetables couldn't be separated from my whiteness and my presumed wealth. Bringing vegetables inadvertently framed our conversations as about health, while food gifts opened up different kinds of conversations.

# 5 · EMBODIED ANALYTICS

the faasamoa is perfect they sd
from behind cocktail bars like pulpits
double scotch on the rocks, I sd

we have no orphans, no one starves
we share everything they sd
refill my glass, I sd

and we all have alofa
for one another, they sd
drown me in your alofa then, I sd

its true they sd, our samoa
is a paradise, we venerate our royalty
our pastors and leaders and beloved dead
god gave us the faasamoa and
only he can take it away, they sd
amen, I sd

their imported first class whisky
was alive with corpses; my uncle
and his army of hungry kids
malnutritioned children in dirty wards
an old woman begging in the bank
my generation migrating overseas
for jobs, while politicians and merchants brag obesely
in the RSA[1] and pastors bang
out sermons about the obedient
and righteous life—aiafu
all growing fat in a blind man's paradise
                    —(Wendt 1976; quoted in
                       Schoeffel 1994, 372–372)[2]

Television on Sundays in Samoa is all church, and so after church services and lunch were complete, Tanu and I would lie on pandanus mats and listen to sermons and to church choirs. One afternoon, I asked him about the women's choir we were watching—two rows of women in white puletasi and hats with hymnals singing *O oe o le Tupu Moni* ("You are the True King"). Tanu squinted, "You don't know they are faletua?" He said they were the wives of the pastors in training in the mainline church. "That's why they are so fat. Imagine what will happen when they find churches!" Tanu chuckled as he continued to watch the choir. This was quite early in my fieldwork, and it was only later that I came to realize that the clothing (e.g., white dress, white hat) and hymnals, not their body size, identified these women. However, Tanu thought their body size was a more important indicator, and certainly a better jibe.

This jovial conversation is representative of common instances where body size indicated status or fat indicated an office, like that of pastor. Once, for example, when attending a funeral, I asked a friend to identify the pastor and she quickly pointed out "the fat one." Similarly, Tanu linked the women's status with their body size, and he chided that they would grow fatter once they had churches to call home. His comments were both humorous and mundane. Tanu's humor rested on my ignorance: how could I not see the obvious meaning of their big bodies? However, humor also rested in the unimaginably quick pace with which pastors and their wives were expected to grow fat once they were placed in churches. "Imagine what will happen when they find churches!" It was expected that the women would grow fat because their congregations would give "their best" to the pastor and his family. The joke also begged the question: would their fat be well deserved?

Criticisms of leadership, as evident in Wendt's poem in the epigraph to this chapter, are not new. Wendt contrasts the wealth of pastors (they drink expensive whiskey) with the poverty of his family ("malnutritioned kids") as a way to draw attention to inequalities generated from reciprocity. While the ideals of fa'asamoa revolve around sharing—there are "no orphans, no one starves, we share everything"—Wendt uses fat to depict the negative side of fa'asamoa. When he writes, "politicians and merchants brag obesely" and these leaders and pastors grow "fat in a blind man's paradise," he suggests that corrupt power is visible in largess in action and body. While scholarly accounts of Samoa often highlight the importance of fa'aaloalo, ethnographers have also noted an equally strong Samoan ambivalence toward endemic hierarchies defined by the ideals of fa'aaloalo. This ambivalence is evident in two sets of conflicting values operating in everyday life. On the one hand, there is a "set of Samoan values emphasizing cooperation, harmony, deference to authority, and the subordination of antisocial impulses to the needs of the group" (Shore 1990, 170). In Tanu's joke, this set of values is evident in the assumption that congregations will give abundantly to the pastor and his family—making them fat. However, "another set of Samoan values emphasiz(es) personal heroism, boldness, competitiveness, fierce loyalty to one's own group" (Shore 1990, 170). Similarly, in Tanu's joke, the assumption is that congregants will give competitively to give the best. In the following pages, I explore how fat talk—everyday talk about fat that creates patterned social relations—expresses these ambivalences in ways that draw attention to conventional hierarchies in churches.

Fat is a material that lends itself to these kinds of discussions, because, in Samoa, there are multiple meanings of fatness. On the one hand, fat is good, especially for women, babies, and old people. On the other, increasingly, fat is thought to be bad because it introduces risk of cardiometabolic disorders. This polyvalence also reflects conflicting ideas about wealth and responsibility. On the one hand, Samoan people are expected to give to their extended families and churches, and large-scale exchange events are an example of how relationships between families are solidified through the exchange of gifts. On the other hand, people need to be able to provide for the nuclear family as distinct from the extended family. References to fat were a way to talk about these competing demands, as fat could indicate both social embeddedness and individual accumulation. In this context, fat talk is commentary about the distribution of resources, forming an embodied analytics. These analytics provided Pentecostals with a way to interpret the signs of the body (e.g., fat, thin, sick, weak, strong) as indicators of how people used their wealth, revealing a Pentecostal ethics of wealth. "Everywhere human conduct is pervaded by an ethical dimension," James Laidlaw writes, "by questions of the rightness and wrongness of actions, or what we owe to each other, of the kind of person we think we are or aspire to be" (2013, 1). I use the term "ethics of wealth" to focus on everyday practices of evaluation and how claims about good bodies are often claims about good wealth. This mode of evaluation draws from the Samoan logic of *mana* (sacred power), where body size can index wealth and power, positioning the body as a mediator between god/s and humans.[3] Fat talk about pastors generated differences between "good bodies" and "bad bodies" in ways that helped Pentecostals evaluate the differences between "good wealth" and "bad wealth."

## EMBODIED ANALYTICS

Interpreting fat is not a static semiotic operation—fat does not automatically mean sick, rich, poor, or stupid.[4] Fat requires context for interpretation, and Pentecostals weaved together threads of information—ranging from whether a pastor worked his own plantation to how he used food gifts—to interpret fat. I look to fat talk to show how Pentecostals connected seemingly disparate wealth practices and theories of power into an interpretive framework for discerning cardiometabolic risk. Fat talk about pastors did not valorize or stigmatize fat, but instead helped people to talk about power by making visible, as people's bodies changed size, the social context in which some people had more access to wealth and power than others.

Mimi Nichter first developed the term fat talk to describe her work with adolescent girls in the United States. She defined fat talk as a "pervasive speech performance" that "facilitates social relations" (Nichter 2000, 4). For example, when adolescent girls made statements like, "I'm so fat," they prompted peers to reassure them that they were not fat. More recently, Greenhalgh defined fat talk as "communication of all sorts about weight—spoken words, written texts, visual images, and moving videos—along with the associated practices, such as dieting, exercising, and many others" (2015, 6). Greenhalgh argues that fat talk is a form of discipline, creating fat subjects even among people who may not be overweight or obese. The pervasiveness of fat talk among young people in the United States creates weight-obsessed citizens, which can be damaging for health. The experience of stigma, generated from feeling like one lives in an environment that doesn't fit their body or around weight-based language, negatively impacts health while increasing suffering (Brewis et al. 2016; Trainer, Brewis, Williams, et al. 2015; Trainer et al. 2016; Taylor 2017).

Fat talk is also endemic to Christian approaches to weight loss. Pentecostal movements like "Pray the Weight Away" or diet gurus like Gwen Shamblin, who famously claimed, "Fat people don't go to heaven," crystalize "profound ambivalence about the flesh" (Griffith 2004, 23).[5] R. Marie Griffith captures the enduring quality of this ambivalence when she writes, "Monks wasting away in the desert, saints beating their bodies and sleeping on nails, apostles renouncing all pleasures and subsisting on the charity of benefactors, pious men and women starving their senses in emulation of Christ" all demonstrate how the body is a "burden that must be suffered resignedly during earthly life" (2004, 23). Fat talk is one way that Christians manage the everyday contradictions around understanding the body as both a source of constant temptation and the site for achieving salvation. For example, among white middle-class Americans in the late 1800s, the thin body was situated as the ideal medium to achieving devotional intimacy (Griffith 2004, 161).[6] On the other hand, among nuns in Mexico, the body needs to be disciplined through sexual abstention and fasting as a way to achieve intimacy with God (Lester 2005). In both examples, the Christian stance toward the body is one of denial. This sense of denial contrasts Samoan ideas about the body, where food consumption has historically been linked to experiences of community care.

In Oceania, bodies make the social efforts of their communities visible. Bodies reflect the fecundity of the land and related community wealth through everyday practices of exchange—the sharing of cash, food, and other resources. In her study of the body in Fiji, Becker finds that "the cumulative efforts of . . . caregivers are embodied in the morphology of their charges" (1995, 57). It is worth pausing to reflect on the word "charges"—the body is not one's own, but rather, a community achievement. Thus, the community, not the individual, is responsible for the care of the body. The body, however, does not just signify in an outward fashion (i.e., the body is a sign interpreted by a community of others) but is also a site for "empirical validation" for the self (Tengan 2008, 87). Writing of Hawai'i, Ty Kawika Tengan draws from the Hawaiian educator Manulani Meyer to explain how bodily experience is a mode of learning. Meyer writes, "Knowing something is feeling something" and "is metaphorically housed in our stomach region because that is also the site of our emotions, our wisdom, as if knowledge also shapes how we emote" (Meyer quoted in Tengan 2008, 87). In this sense, it is possible to understand how the body, and the stomach in particular, mediates individual experience and social life, and thereby indicates authority derived from knowledge and relationships. For men in Samoa, the stomach was also the focus of attentive criticism.

The body is, therefore, a site of experience and a symbol that indicates the relationship between self and community. Accordingly, qualities of the body, like slowness, fatness, or sleepiness, can indicate the relationships that produce those experiences (Munn 1986, 17). From this perspective, the body is symbolic of the relationships that help to produce it. In Samoa, the relationships between family members or between families, for example, create food—through laboring on plantations, gift giving, or sharing food from a single pot—and make it possible for some people to be fat. In this way, the body indicates the functioning of social units. However, as the food environment changes, so too do the ways in which people relate around and through food. Simply put, as Samoans purchase more food than they grow themselves, they can access dense amounts of fat, which was otherwise reserved for only a few. Those few who had access to fat were thought to be situated within dense social networks—saying things like, "they have strong families." However, as more people can access more calories, being fat does not necessarily mean that one is at the center of a dense social network—saying things like, "they don't have land," or people are "lazy." Having a lot of food might instead indicate access to a few wealthy family members or a prestigious job—singular nodes in a family network. As a result, there are multiple meanings of fatness, and in turn, people needed ways to determine if fat was created through community sharing or individual selfishness. By only looking at body size, one could not tell the difference. Fat talk, about pastors, was one way to evaluate this difference. Talking about fat was, therefore, a way to talk about social and economic difference.

In turn, fat talk is a kind of valuation, the practices of creating and ranking differences and "deciding what kinds of differences are important" (Ferry 2013, 18; see also Gregory 1997, 13). Embodied analytics refers to the ways that fat talk is a mode of valuation that collapses distinctions between economic, embodied, and religious spheres. In Samoa, fat talk compares fat in unlike forms—adipose tissue, fatty cuts of meat, fat in canned foods—with the social practices that generate those forms of fat—that is, working a plantation, giving food gifts at a funeral, or providing meals to pastors. Elsewhere in Oceania, as in Samoa, practices like sharing and giving foods, or other valuables, are part of what makes them valuable. Annette Weiner (1992) described this phenomenon as the paradox of keeping-while-giving, where gifts may be given away, but always maintain some connection to the giver. While gift exchange is predicated on always giving objects—like food, textiles, or the armbands and necklaces of kula, the objects cannot be alienated, or separated, from the giver or the history of their giving (see also Young 1972). Writing of Palau, Richard Parmentier writes, "Movement and stasis actually imply each other: to generate its exchange value, *udoud* [Palauan money] must travel, yet to accomplish its maximal work, it must be kept long enough in contiguity with some social unit to become identified with it" (2002, 65). Holding on to money for too long, however, could also make one vulnerable to curses (Parmentier 2002, 65–66). Pentecostals, similarly, linked pastoral sickness with wealth that wasn't given away; wealth that pastors held on to had the potential to make those pastors sick and so revealed how stationary wealth could be a source of bodily decay.

From this perspective, wealth that did not move between God, leaders, and the community could be risky, both socially and to one's health. On the one hand, fat was beneficial when the large body was the "outcome" of the movement of resources (see Munn 1986). On the other hand, the fat body that did not mediate between social spheres became an indicator of individual wealth, which was rendered suspect (see Bohannan 1955). Nancy Munn shows the mediating role of the body in exchange relationships: "For instance, if Gawans eat a great deal instead of giving food to overseas visitors, they fail to create the kind of overseas expansion of self made possible through hospitality. Instead of outward, self-extending acts, their acts are, in effect, self-focused, since they involve the incorporation of their own food, and in Gawan terms, the "disappearance" of the food and thus any further potentialities it may have for positive transformations" (1986, 13).

Here Munn is talking about the ways food becomes an extension of the self, entering the bodies of others as a way of expanding social influence. In an analogous way, the examples to follow suggest that Pentecostals considered fat healthy, and a sign of strength, when the fat person was known to give generously. However, fat was risky when the person was thought to be greedy. Risk and health were, therefore, inextricably tied to how one used resources. Fat was considered both positive (i.e., indicating that one was on the receiving end of many relationships) and suspect (i.e., indicating the potential that the person was not moving those resources into other relationships). Fat was a malleable sign because it indicated both wealth that was shared *and* wealth that was consumed. Pentecostals might wonder: How many cans of corned beef did that pastor eat last night? Where did those cans come from? By extension, how do you know what fat is good, what fat makes one strong, and what fat is bad and makes one sick?

## CHURCH OFFERINGS: COMPETITION
## AND INSTITUTIONAL NORMS

A self-proclaimed former "9 AM Catholic" (i.e., a Catholic in name only, who only attends morning Mass to be seen by others), Tai, who was in her forties, was newly born again. She felt she had been "forced to become like them to be part of that group" in her Catholic church; she felt she had to participate in competitive giving to be accepted by the congregation, many of whom were also her family. She felt the most important part of her church participation was "how much I could give in my offering," which meant that she could not "feel any joy in church, just obligation": "There's too much emphasis on what other people think, rather than what God thinks. To look good in front of others, to look strong, to look wealthy, to be accomplished, and of course when the pastor praises them, the congregants bestow favors on him. So a lot of them are thinking of man rather than Him." Tai pointed upward.

Tai felt alienated by the pressures to perform, while she also questioned the fact that gifts were used as the primary measure of moral worth, generosity, and commitment to family. She thought that people attended church mostly to impress the pastor, not "to be with God."

Gifts indicated the wealth of congregations, and therefore the families that historically practiced within those villages. When traveling to Samoa for the first time, a taxi driver asked me if I knew which houses were for the pastors. I declined, not yet knowing how to read village landscapes. He said, "They are the only houses with two storeys." Cars, houses, home furnishings, and church architecture did not directly indicate the prestige of the pastor, but pointed instead to the wealth, service, and generosity of the families within the congregation. This tradition is derived from missionary strategies to embed Christianity into Samoan culture. When villages decided to accept Christianity, they built a church and a house for the teacher or the pastor and his family. The village began to contribute to the church, supporting the mission with food and services. Families contributed coconut oil and arrowroot starch to the mission, which was shipped to England for sale to raise money for the mission (Meleisea 1987). The missionaries also introduced the custom of making public church donations; before people had money to give, family leaders would call out the amount of oil their family had made for the church. Historically, then, families, villages, and districts "competed for the honor of giving the most to the church" (Meleisea 1987, 55). This legacy continues today as there was constant pressure to give (often, as much as possible) to the church, making commitment to the church *sin qua non* commitment to family.[7] One pastor explained on a TV news segment that the "authority of the church" comes from the annual conference, which is also the most significant fundraiser of the year.

The realities of these pressures were made clear to me through weekly conversations with Ferila, a newly born-again single mother in her late thirties. She often talked about the "stress" of budgeting for her household: utilities, food, church, and family offerings. Jokingly, she explained, she gave her mother as little as she could for church offerings because she knew her mother would give as much as possible. "I always know if mum is grouchy it's because she doesn't have enough for the church offering," she teased. With laughter and a raised eyebrow, she continued, "Our kitchen cupboards would be empty!" Iterating Christian prosperity ideas, Ferila was excited to learn about the "benefit of the believer," which meant she could "command her kitchen cupboards full when mom gave everything to the pastor."

I start this section with Tai and Ferila because their reflections highlight some of the key ways that Pentecostals criticized community giving: competition, the prioritization of public representations of the family reputation over family needs, and the presence of the pastor as a source of social pressure. These critiques make sense within the cultural context of Samoa where competition is palpable and church-based giving is extensively organized. Mainline churches require weekly or fortnightly cash offerings to support the pastor and his family, including rent-free residence, land to grow food crops, free labor to maintain that land and household, payment of utilities, and vehicle maintenance (Macpherson and Macpherson 2011, 315). Pastors also receive gifts for participating in weddings, funerals, blessings at new constructions, or baptisms, in addition to annual gifts.[8] During these times of year, the shops in town hold massive sales, advertising in print and on the radio. These annual events generate competition not only within the congregation but also between villages. In 2010, for example, in one village, thirteen Congregational churches provided luxury vehicles for their pastors' use, which ranged from $76,950 to $145,000 tālā (Macpherson and Macpherson 2011).[9] When pastors receive particularly expensive cars, they are often featured in the newspaper, making their villages well known across the islands. In addition to these regular obligations, church members support occasional church construction projects, personal gifts for pastors' sabbaticals, retirements and medical treatments, or wedding and graduation gifts for family of the pastor (Macpherson and Macpherson 2011, 321). Part of the reason pastors maintain such an important role in daily life reflects missionization efforts to attribute the sacred power of chiefs to pastors. In pre-Christian Samoa, "the highest chiefs could do almost anything they wished, so great was the mana they received from the gods" (Meleisea 1987, 68). With Christianity, matai maintained their "divinely inspired authority," but this power was thought to be derived instead from a single Christian God (Meleisea 1987, 69). Pastors were also thought to derive their authority from this single Christian God. Even hundreds of years later, it is not hard to see how millions of Samoan tālā circulate on any given Sunday (Macpherson and Macpherson 2011).

Pentecostal churches practice tithing, in contrast, and they position this as the opposite of gift-based offerings. There are two main ways that tithing is represented as different. First, it is private. When the amount is recorded, it is not connected to particular family names as the treasurer often does in mainline churches. The tithe amount is never announced, as mainline churches tend to. Second, the tithe is considered fairer because it is a percentage of earnings, so families who earn different amounts each pay 10 percent. If the family doesn't earn any cash, but instead are subsistence farmers, they can contribute 10 percent of their agricultural products or their labor to the church, not the pastor. In the next sections, I highlight three examples of fat talk that serve as critical commentary on church giving as the opposite of tithing and how fat helps to construct this opposition.

## PREACHING ABOUT FAT

On a Sunday morning in Apia, Pastor Sefo started his sermon by stating, "Many will be called but few will be chosen." Pacing the stage, Pastor Sefo asked the congregation to open their Bibles to the Book of Matthew to focus his sermon on the difficulties of practicing a "Christian life." Aiming to make his sermon relatable, Pastor Sefo told a story of his recent trip to Savai'i, the rural "big" island of Samoa, where he met an old friend who was also a Pentecostal pastor. As they chatted, they became hungry, and when they docked in Savai'i, they decided to eat. Pastor Sefo said, "Of course we went to visit our old friend, a Congregational pastor." The congregants chuckled, already picking up on the implication of Pastor Sefo's statement, when he said, "The pastor's house is where all the food is, eh?" The congregants laughed heartily, responding emphatically, "hallelujah" and "that's true." The taken-for-granted assumption in this joke was that pastors were free from want—their congregations cared for their needs, and to arrive at the pastor's house was to eat good food. Joking about this in a knowing way, Pastor Sefo suggested that even as a pastor, he would take advantage of this abundance on occasion.

Pastor Sefo was young, perhaps in his early forties, known as a former rugby player; he wore slim-fitting shirts to accentuate his muscularity. In his story, he embodied youth and strength when depicting himself and the other Pentecostal pastor. He threw his shoulders back, puffed out his chest, and took broad steps, miming a broad and strong body as he paced to one side of the stage to "meet" the mainline pastor. He brought the congregation further in by switching from the signs of youthful virility to humbleness to depict how he and his friend waited for the mainline pastor to emerge from his private room. His exaggerated humbleness—turned shoulders inward, gaze upward—suggested that the office of mainline pastor demanded that they perform respect. Through his imitations, Pastor Sefo contrasted the mainline and Pentecostal pastors. He depicted the mainline pastor sitting alone, not in the common social areas of the house. He highlighted the social isolation of the mainline pastor resulting from this performance of respect. In contrast, he exaggerated the ideal of Pentecostal egalitarianism when narrating his interaction with his friend, the Pentecostal pastor, with whom he informally joked (see also Eriksen 2014).

When Pastor Sefo switched to narrating the mainline pastor, he imitated sickness and fatness. He mimed an old man—taking small steps, hunching his shoulders, slowly dragging his feet toward his two friends from youth. This mainline pastor, he explained, was very "big," and sick with gout. He rounded his arms and pointed his elbows away from his body to directly link disease, body size, and food abundance. He then read from the Book of Matthew: "Then Jesus said to his disciples, 'Truly I tell you, it is hard for someone who is rich to enter the Kingdom of Heaven. Again I tell you, it is easier for a camel to go through the eye of a needle than for someone who is rich to enter the Kingdom of God.'" By connecting this scripture with contrasting images of youthful Pentecostal pastors and a fat/sick mainline pastor, Pastor Sefo taught congregants to understand fatness and sickness as suspiciously interrelated signs.

This brief section of a Sunday morning sermon shows how Pentecostals make fat meaningful by looking to wealth. Congregants learned that wealth that was generated by obligation, as was the assumed case with the mainline pastor, created sickness. Pastor Sefo represented the pastor's body as a social body, which Nancy Scheper-Hughes and Margaret Lock have famously defined as a "natural symbol for thinking about relationships among nature, society, and culture" (1987, 6). In this case, the pastor's fat body was a symbol for talking about the relationship between wealth, community, and the body. When Pastor Sefo linked abundant food, fatness, and sickness, he implied that the mainline pastor's wealth was inappropriate because it was given to him without being earned. In other words, abundant resources, like food, were deemed positive insofar as they were redistributed among those who originally provided the resources in the form of gifts. The gifts indicated the strength of the community, and it was the responsibility of the leader to ensure that all those who contributed were provided for as a result. In this case, wealth that did not circulate was unethical. Fat that did not move between leaders and communities was fat that could cause sickness, advanced age, and immobility.

Through this story, the pastor taught his congregants to look at fat in a new way. They were instructed to see connections between fatness, weakness, and sickness and to interpret these signs as indications of dishonesty. On the surface, this interpretation seems to reflect a medicalized idea of fat, where fat is considered a risk factor. However, Pastor Sefo's analysis differed because fat was not risky. The practices that generated the fat (e.g., hoarding resources, not sharing) were the source of risk. Therefore, risk provided a framework where fat and sickness became linked, but the embodied analytics that Pentecostals invoked added another dimension to this framework: the ethics of wealth. Pastor Sefo focused on *how* fat was accumulated in the body as fundamental to understanding *if* the fat was dangerous to health.

## EATING SWEAT, EATING SHEEP

Before her conversion, Telisa said she was accustomed to the pastor's method of "badgering" the congregation for offerings. She believed it was the will of God, as she imagined God to be distant, where pastors had the responsibility to mediate, through whatever means necessary, between congregants and God. However, after conversion, Telisa began to relate to God, and her pastor, in new ways. She began to seek a personal, direct, and reciprocal relationship with God. I learned about her conversion one afternoon as we ate leftovers from the previous night—*kokoraisa* (rice with coconut cream and Samoan cocoa)—while laying on mats on the porch to avoid working up a sweat. Using eating metaphors, Telisa and her husband, Ioane, talked about how they had been struggling to meet the financial obligations of their families. What made their obligations even more onerous was that, in both of their family's churches, they felt alienated.

When Telisa was a teenager, she shared with her pastor that she was sexually active because she felt she "needed to repent and tell the truth." She was looking for "help, to change." Instead of receiving the counsel she sought, the pastor told her not to return to church. For years following this, Telisa continued to contribute to her family's offering but was not welcome to church. She felt she deserved it because she had sinned in an unforgiveable way. When she married Ioane, however, she hoped it would be better in his church. However, Ioane's family treated Telisa more like a "housekeeper than a daughter."[10] Telisa was again expected to stay at home during church services to prepare the to'ona'i, not participating in church services yet still contributing to church offerings.

Feeling lethargic, depressed, and lonely, Telisa met a Pentecostal faletua at a work function and immediately felt like she wanted to get to know her. She eventually made an appointment with her to talk about her struggles with church, and this was the occasion of her conversion. After this, she began attending evening services at that church—services that didn't conflict with her Sunday duties to her husband's family. At this time, she began to feel uncomfortable about contributing to her family's offerings and started to resent the pastor, feeling the offerings he solicited showed that he was selfish and greedy. Sometimes, when she would sneak into the back of the church hall, she would hear him preach in ways that made her feel she had to give the most to show her alofa to God.

After spending a few months attending evening services at a Pentecostal church where the faletua pastored, Telisa invited Ioane to join her. On the first evening he attended, he was born again because he felt "the Spirit of God opened and changed [his] heart." For the first time, he wanted to go to church "to fellowship with God and listen to the Word and to do what the Bible says and tithe." He immediately connected conversion with giving in a new way, a way that was standardized and not based on the expectations set by the pastor, but a perceived universal directive from the Bible.

Telisa and Ioane both narrated their conversion through a discussion of changed giving practices, and even more, once they converted, they spent a great deal of time learning the "truth" in the Bible about giving—reciting biblical passages as evidence of this "truth." Telisa favored Malachi 3:8: "Will a mere mortal rob God? Yet you rob me. But you ask, 'How are we robbing you?' In tithes and offerings." She learned how to interpret this verse in her new church, where it was used to suggest that, when one didn't tithe, they were not only absconding their duty to God, but were also stealing from God. In the mainline church, she said, "the people believe when they give money to the pastor they are giving money to God, but they just don't understand. [The pastors] turn the Bible upside down to spread their message about *meaalofa* (gifts/offerings)." Skeptically, Telisa felt pastors were seeking to increase offerings from congregants as a way to increase their own wealth. Tithing was considered a just way for individuals to calculate their offering in standard and shared ways that did not require the pastor to weigh in. "The church should give to people instead of the people, who have nothing, giving to the pastor, who is already," she paused and mimed a fat stomach by raising her elbows to her sides, "you know?" Linking wealth with a fat stomach, Telisa implied that the pastors were wealthy at the expense of the congregants.

As Telisa finished speaking, Ioane urgently added, "Sometimes people are eating only taro because they have given all their money and food to the pastor." As I discussed earlier, ideally, everyone living on family land should have access to starch staples like taro. To say someone eats "only taro" is to say the family is unable to afford the basic accompaniments to starchy foods, like meat, that make a meal complete. Those who lived in urban areas of Apia, however, often did not have access to land and so were more cash dependent than those who could grow their own food. This was the case for Telisa and Ioane. "The people are hungry," Ioane said, "and they don't have anything, no money." And yet, he concluded, "the pastor is fat." This prototype suggested that pastors were fat because they "*'ai afu* [eat the sweat] of the people." This metaphor, *'ai afu*, suggested that pastors took advantage of their authority and consumed without limits while congregants experienced deprivation as a result. The congregants were "working but the pastor gets everything for free" in an unequal exchange or by unfulfilled reciprocity. Congregants gave but did not receive in return. Congregants were, therefore, compelled to participate in one-way gifting rather than exchange, and were economically insecure as a result—they skipped meals, they were hungry, spiritually and physically. This contrasted with the ways this spiritual economy was expected to work, where pastors mediated between God and the congregation, thereby bringing forth prosperity into the community.

Ioane extended the eating metaphor when he capped off his critique with an accusation that pastors "*'ai mamoe* [eat sheep] too." Using the biblical metaphor of the shepherd, he continued, "eating the sheep he should be leading." When I asked Ioane to explain, he said, sometimes pastors have affairs with girls in the village. This is a grave accusation, but one I had heard before in stories of "bad" pastors. Ioane used this metaphor to create a composite of pastors who used congregants' bodies as resources to sate individual appetites. He represented this composite pastor as taking from his congregants while also violating the morals he likely espoused in Sunday sermons. The contrast between what pastors preached and their everyday behaviors was particularly important to many Pentecostals I knew. They often focused on how these pastors were not "role models" for youth because of their consumption, often smoking and drinking alcohol. Though not Pentecostal, the poem that opens this chapter highlights, in a sarcastic tone, the contrast between what leaders say and what they do—"we share everything they sd . . . we all have alofa for one another."

The centrality of the word 'ai (to eat) illuminates the importance of consumption as a way to talk about wealth, health, and reproduction. "To eat," as Elizabeth Wende Marshall (2012a; 2012b) and Valerio Valeri (1985) note of Hawai'i, does not "begin to approach the multivalent depth of the cluster of Hawaiian concepts centered on 'ai" (Marshall 2012a, 71). Valeri translates 'ai as commensal—to refer to the ways that organisms benefit from one another—contrasting this to simple consumption (1985, 104). This expansiveness extends to Samoa, where eating is both an action and a concept, mediating the relationship between people and spirits through the transformation of things—like land and food generated from that land—in the body. The examples of eating sweat and sheep suggested power that was uncontrolled. While the power of pastors has typically been associated with the generation of prosperity for the community, these metaphors drew attention to how power generated individual wealth, not community prosperity. Fat talk was, therefore, a way to evaluate the quality of the relationship between congregants and pastors.

## FAT MEN IN WHITE BLAZERS

One weekday, before the household started bustling with early-morning activities, I found Lagi sleeping on the couch. Later, she explained that she stayed awake until 5 AM writing about a vision she had of "the counterfeit."[11] From Lagi's perspective, counterfeits were replicas of people that looked and acted like real people but, instead, were demonic imitations of real people. During her office-based prayer group, Lagi had her first vision of a counterfeit. This was an image of a "pale fat man" wearing a white 'iefaitaga (men's formal lāvalava) and a white blazer. Every Sunday, mainline church-goers wear their bleached, starched, and ironed white clothing; women wear elaborate hats, while men wear white 'iefaitaga. Typically, only pastors or other church elders wear white blazers, so the blazer that Lagi imagined served as a symbol of mainstream Christianity, while the paleness indicated physical weakness. She later wrote in her journal a message that accompanied her vision that the Holy Spirit communicated to her: "One, the end is coming, two, Christians are refusing Christ, and three, there is a need for a new group of priests and evangelists to do the warfare needed."[12]

Lagi continued to elaborate on her vision of the fat, pale pastor over the next few weeks in her prayer meetings. The next day, Lagi shared with her office-based prayer group how she interpreted her vision: "unsaved" leaders in churches and the government were having a negative impact on the island, causing increased sickness and suffering. She reminded her peers, Samoa was a country "founded upon God's word," and as a result, "people receive blessings in everything through its leaders." Like Ioane, she felt Samoans were vulnerable as long as its leaders were not saved. "There is great darkness at the top," meaning the nation's leaders were not saved and "in the dark regarding God's will." Instead of judging them, she told the group, "we should pray and uplift these leaders to Him." All the group could do was pray so that God could "work on the things that we uplift." The group was responsible for "standing together in love and with humble hearts before Him."[13] She ended with a brief prayer: "Lord, please Father, let not your wrath come upon our people because of these leaders."

Lagi saw herself as actively working against these kinds of leaders in her prayer group. She was "given the word 'separation'" by the Holy Spirit with the accompanying message to "chaff that what has already been separated from the wheat, it is the harvest." Drawing from a millennialist metaphor of the harvest, Lagi articulated that she saw a separation between current leadership and an emerging cadre of prayer warriors, who were responsible for separating the chaff (waste) from wheat. When Lagi started to think about this message, she felt that since the end was near, "we must work, we must pray for our country for our people." Most importantly, she beseeched the group, "We must stand together to pray to Him for he is a Father who is full of love. He will hear us, but we have to do our job, together, stand together and make it a practice now every day to stand together for the righteousness of God to prevail in our spiritual leaders."

Lagi's vision of the pale, fat pastor clearly placed the office of pastor in question—drawing attention to how leaders can negatively impact the well-being of the broader community. She interpreted this fat pastor as a "false prophet" who was one of the "biggest challenges for Christians today." These false prophets encouraged Christians to perform faith on Sundays, and to make offerings an essential part of that performance, but in their "hearts," Lagi feared, they were not "living by the Word of God." As with other examples in this chapter, Lagi focused on the problem of giving. In her mentoring of other women, Lagi often prompted them to question the authority of pastors. During one of Lagi's Bible study groups, Amataga, a recently born-again woman in her late thirties, expressed some difficulties she faced when visiting her mother's mainline church. When she went to the Mother's Day church services in her village, she said, "The devil got the best of me. My mom only had fifty tālā, and here I am coming from Apia. So I said here, put a hundred."[14] After, Amataga said to herself, "This is why I don't want to come to this church anymore." Lagi comforted her: "Well that's what the church does to you. It compels you to do things." Lagi also communicated this idea when she would jokingly call mainstream church offerings a "cover charge," as if the money paid was to enter a nightclub. Here, she focused on how the church, as a social institution, compelled action in ways that challenged an individual's ability to connect with God, while the tithe was a private obligation to God, a biblical obligation.[15]

## FAT ETHICS

Fat talk communicated that when wealth was distributed in unethical ways, it could cause sickness. According to this logic, leaders were responsible for redistributing wealth to allow for blessings to flow from leader to community—an idea shared across Christianities. However, when Pentecostals engaged in fat talk, they created an ethics of wealth that used fat as a measure of well-being. This ethics of wealth suggested that pastors should provide for congregants, not the other way around. When leaders did not redistribute wealth, congregants suffered— financially, emotionally, and physically. Fat was a particularly illustrative material to make this critique because the body changed in size, shape, and health in ways that could be explained in relation to wealth. Talking about wealth through discussions of fat thus provided embodied evidence to substantiate social critiques.

According to this critique, when pastors failed to act as conduits between the heavens and the earth, their fatness could be interpreted as a sign of sickness, not prosperity. Here stagnant wealth materialized in sickness, whereas ethical wealth moved between spheres of sacred and human. This movement between spheres created big and strong bodies. Fat talk critiqued pastors for the ways that they wielded wealth/power and suggested that this made them sick. As a result, fat talk about powerful community leaders brought into question taken-for-granted assumptions about reciprocity. In this way, fat talk was performative—through speaking about fat, the expectations of responsibility between pastors and congregants were transformed.[16] Feminist theorist Judith Butler has expanded how scholars think about performativity to include ways that discourse creates relationships through repeated speech. The "reiterative power of discourse," she writes, produces "the phenomena that it regulates and constrains" (Butler 1993, 2). In other words, discourse reflects reality while regulating what is considered normal. Fat talk is one such regulatory discourse, shaping how body size norms are experienced. In the United States, for example, fat talk is also often "epidemic talk," where thinness is "imbued with the rationality and self-discipline of perfect subjects" and fatness brings into question the "deservingness" of citizens (Guthman and DuPuis 2006, 427).

Pentecostal fat talk about pastors, in contrast, reflected anxieties about hierarchy and reciprocity—creating moral messages about community through moral messages about wealth. Rather than blaming individuals, fat talk communicated that unethical wielding of power/wealth could enhance risk for cardiometabolic sickness. While fat was increasingly associated with risk, it was not the material itself that was risky, but the ways that fat was attained—through particular choices around wealth distribution or accumulation. While value creation depends on ranking and creating differences between particular objects, value also refers to the "invisible chains that link relations between things to relations between people" (Gregory 1997, 13). Through fat talk, Pentecostals called into question these invisible links between people. Embodied analytics encouraged Pentecostals to view the body as a source of evidence for understanding how leaders distributed resources. In other words, the body's symptoms, like numbness, sores, or blindness—all complications related to diabetes—were evidence of how wealth was accumulated and distributed. Through fat talk, Pentecostals learned how to interpret this evidence in ways that scaled up their etiologies, from individual suffering to social suffering caused by inequalities felt from serving conventional hierarchies.

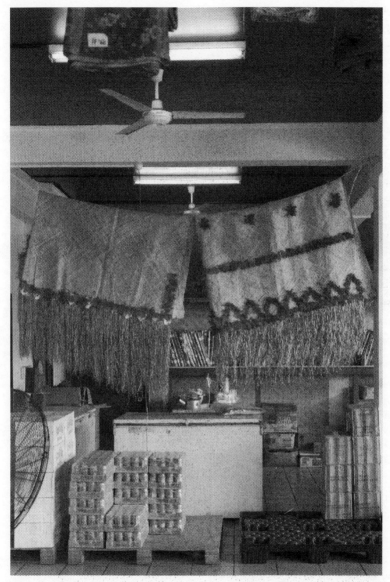

FIGURE 9 Two women sit fanning themselves in one of the shops that strictly focuses on suppling fa'alavelave needs in Apia. I peeked my head in and whispered, asking if I could take a photo. The younger woman turned to the older woman, and the older woman raised her eyebrow and nodded in my direction. The *'ie tōga* (fine mats) were eye-catching from the window. These fine mats, once objects that gained their value from the months of work that women would invest in weaving soft, detailed pandanus, were now sold in markets across Samoa. The shop sells the items that are absolutely required for participation in fa'alavelave including fine mats, fizzy drinks, frozen meat, and boxes of tinned fish or corned beef, bolts of fabric. When I first started fieldwork in Samoa these shops were rare, as these items were integrated into larger markets. Now markets were specializing.

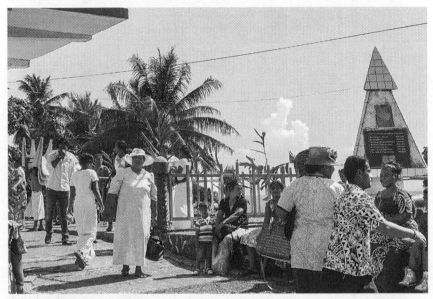

FIGURE 10 The church was decorated with leaves and flowers because this was a special Sunday, the last service in the church before it would be torn down to build another in its place. When the service ended, there was a hustle of activity as rows of chairs were arranged around tables that emerged from the pastor's house. Young people began scurrying between the kitchen and the church with trays of food—first serving bowls of ice cream, then plates of rice, noodles, taro, and chicken. Platters were distributed to the elders and prestigious visitors, including other pastors and matai. The congregation had collected enough money to rebuild the pastor's house, which was across the road, and still under construction. They were close to their goal to rebuild the church, so they started disassembling it. Until the church was rebuilt, they would have their services in the church hall, also across the road, an open-air building that seemed to touch the ocean. Congregants were proud to be able to build a new home for the pastor and his family and a new church, but they were also proud to tell me how little it was costing. Their budget was modest when compared to other recent church building projects, which seemed decadent. Hundreds of people came to this farewell service to commemorate their family's contribution to church, old and new.

# 6 · WELL-BEING AND DEFERRED AGENCY

Kika, a physician in her early forties who was living with diabetes, told me she was 260 pounds at her heaviest but she lost 40 pounds after recovering from knee surgery.[1] She spent most of the time while recovering stationary, watching Trinity Broadcasting Network (an American Christian television network briefly available in Samoa), and during this time, she was born again. She interpreted her newfound interest in Christian television as a sign that something was "changing" in her: "One afternoon, I was watching a service and the preacher made an altar call for people who wanted to be born again. That's what I did, right from my living room." That's also when she began to feel her "body [was] a living sacrifice." Kika lost weight and learned to "control" her diabetes: "The change I knew couldn't come from myself. I had to pray. I really had to pray. I prayed to God to give me the strength, so I thank God that he gave me the strength and then I was able to stop myself from wanting to eat all the time and the only exercise I did was walking on the seawall."

Kika began to pray for strength and fortitude to continue to "keep [her] healthy lifestyle going." Specifically, she said when she did not turn to "Father" in instances when she did not have the physical strength to exercise or the cash to purchase "vegetables and healthy foods," she heard God whisper, "Why not let me handle that?" Another woman, also a physician, would tell me she was praying for God to move mountains in her life—these mountains were her weaknesses in "the flesh," and she was praying for the strength to change her diet and exercise habits. In still another instance, one faith healer advised a man in the hospital, recovering from amputation surgery, to have courage. Saying, "I cannot bear your pain, only you can and your relationship with God can heal that pain," she reminded him that "through Him you will find solace and comfort so that you may receive healing that only comes from God. Now that you believe in Him, draw close to Him in prayer. We must pray earnestly, without ceasing."

These kinds of intersections emerged all the time in my discussions with people, as instances when health practices were interpreted through the lens of

Pentecostal ideas about wellness. Stories recounting illness and conversion experiences, healing prayers, and salvation prayers during hospital stays all provide viewpoints from which to understand how religious change—that is, being born again—was measured through health. Here I draw a distinction between health and wellness to foreground how the everyday management of food and fat required learning a new set of health techniques around weight management, diet, physical activity, and pharmaceutical use.[2]

Cardiometabolic disorders require those living with them to develop an awareness of health that is metric-centric, attending to how sugar, fat, and salt affect weight, glucose, and blood pressure.[3] Adopting a metric-centric notion of food, fat, and fitness—what Yates-Doerr (2015) calls metrification—privileges the universally derived metric norms of cardiometabolic health—body mass index, blood glucose levels, blood pressure—as key indicators of health at the expense of situational contexts like relationships, environment, and enduring inequalities that shape health. These health techniques include being mindful of nutritional intake—that is, learning to see foods like taro, chicken, potato chips, or cucumbers in terms of nutritional elements like sugar, fat, salt, or nutrients and vitamins (Yates-Doerr 2012b; see also Biltekoff 2013). Health techniques also include seeing the body as a system regulated by inputs and outputs—30 minutes of exercise is a way to balance caloric intake. Health metrics did not play a large role in everyday life in Samoa, as there were no at-home glucometers and body weight scales were not widely available. In clinical environments, however, health practitioners still advised patients in a metric-centric way by encouraging patients to change cardiometabolic metrics—lose weight, reduce sugar and fat intake. These kinds of techniques required individuals to act in ways that foregrounded their individual health efforts, for example, by using resources for medicines or doctor's visits or by changing family meals around individual dietary restrictions. These proved difficult in daily life.

In this chapter, I focus on intersections of Christian conversion and medical events—instances when people were diagnosed or admitted to the hospital because of illness—to provide insight into how deferring to God's agency was a way by which some people changed their health techniques. They placed these practices within a broader effort toward creating Christian wellness. Well-being encompasses biomedical health but is not strictly defined by it and instead refers to a broader set of practices of searching for and cultivating the good life—in this case, how this good life is constructed through Christian moral axioms about consumption and an individually intimate relationship with God. Well-being has also been described as the "ongoing aspiration for something better that gives meaning to life's pursuits," which "involves the arduous work of becoming, of trying to live a life that one deems worthy, becoming the sort of person that one desires" (Fischer 2014, 2). Pentecostalism provides a particular set of practices and ideas aimed at developing a good Christian life—a "range of expressive forms" through which one can learn to develop, as my interlocutors would say, their "walk with Christ" (Klaits 2011, 207). Through these expressive forms, like prayer, "people apprehend their well-being or lack thereof in their own eyes as well as in the views of divine and human others, and through which they perceive how those others have contributed to their welfare or suffering" (Klaits 2011, 207). Scholars have explored how Christian prayer, for example, creates well-being because prayers, as forms of direct communication with God, are often "intended to elicit divine aid" (Corwin 2014, 174). This kind of communication, which can create "a positive interaction with the supernatural," is quite simply "good for people" (Luhrmann 2013, 708).[4] Health science scholars have found that interaction with God about illness experience provides comfort while also often increasing treatment adherence (Stewart et al. 2013). A range of activities, classified as "religious coping," such as prayer, belief that God will provide, and Bible reading, have shown to improve health outcomes, especially for cardiometabolic disorders (Namageyo-Funa and Muilenburg 2013).[5]

Samoan Pentecostal practices, like healing prayers, encouraged those who were born again to come to see health—as both a set of practices and an outcome—as an expression of faith. In general, making changes to everyday health practices around food, fat, and fitness was difficult for most because of the everyday expectations that individuals should place the needs of the family over individual health. Pentecostal notions of well-being, on the other hand, foregrounded individual health as a manifestation of God's will, or the Kingdom of God on earth, encouraging Pentecostals to tend to these health techniques as part of a larger life purpose. Changing health was a way to care for the body as a proxy for cultivating faithfulness to God. However, when Pentecostals represented health as a manifestation of faith, they foregrounded God's work, not individual achievement, in creating that health, thereby deferring individual agency to God's agency. In the examples I explore in this chapter, when people converted during a medical event, their conversion helped them downplay their own motivations for changing health behaviors, and, therefore, through conversion, they were able to de-emphasize individual agency. In these cases, Christian conversion created possible avenues for changing health practices, managing stress, and shifting resource use in the name of religious commitment, which was a creative way for people to manage endemic hierarchies that made changing health behaviors difficult.

## EVERYDAY HEALING

Healing was an everyday occurrence, from the mundane to the extraordinary. Mornings with Lagi often involved ordinary methods. As her kids woke up with bellyaches or headaches, not wanting to go to school, she would lay hands on them and pray over them and send them on their way. I observed more extraordinary healing methods with the healing ministry team of Glory House when they visited the hospital. Before going to the hospital, I would join the group in an empty hall, which on Sundays was the location of the English-speaking congregation, to share church gossip, upcoming travel, or fa'alavelave news. After everyone had arrived, Hana (the ministry leader) would join us and lead a prayer to prepare the group for the work ahead. As the women climbed out of whoever's car was available, they would break into pairs and funnel into the acute ward for visiting hours. I worked with four different women, each of whom had her own style. One was forceful. Another was quiet, and favored listening over preaching. Another liked to ask as many questions as she could, and the last led with humor. In the acute ward, we saw patients ranging in age, injury, and sickness—from a young girl, perhaps twelve years old, who had been hit by a car, to an old man who suffered from asthma. Over half of the men and women the team prayed over were suffering from complications from cardiometabolic disorders. These included sepsis, vision difficulties, chronic wounds, fluid retention, or neuropathy. When the two-hour visitor period was over, the women gathered outside and reported back on how many "souls were saved." One of the elders recorded this number, which was used in ministry reports to church elders. These numbers inevitably created competition among some of the women to "save the most souls." Some, however, ignored this and would spend the entire two hours with one person.

The most common forms of healing I observed were at the end of Sunday services when the pastor would ask anyone who was in need of healing to come to the front of the church for prayer—an altar call. Pastors would move from one person to the next laying on hands and whispering healing prayers into the ears of the supplicant. Congregants and friends would often join in and also lay hands on the supplicant's body. These altar calls were small-scale versions of what would occur during periodic healing services at Glory House. These were either week-long events with visiting preachers from Australia, New Zealand, Fiji, and the United States or single events held during the regularly scheduled Sunday evening services up to four times per year. Healing services usually included a shorter sermon focused on learning healing methods and how to "receive" healing. The pastor would often select an individual from the congregation to come on stage for a "Holy Spirit demonstration." One evening a woman from the healing ministry, Losa, volunteered to touch the pastor's shirt, and as she did, she immediately fell to the ground, mimicking the story in Luke 8:43–48 of a woman who touched Jesus's garment and was immediately healed. She laid on the stage, convulsing, for fifteen minutes before she was ushered off the stage.

After demonstrations, the chairs would be removed and the gym opened up so that the entire congregation—somewhere between one thousand and two thousand people—could crowd the stage to sing worship music. Pastors and their wives, perhaps numbering thirty couples, would encircle the congregation, locking hands and creating a "healing chain." Sometimes pastors would move among the crowds, laying hands on individuals as they were "prompted by the Holy

Spirit," and men and women would be "slain," falling like dominos into the crowd. Other times, the pastors and their wives would stand at the front of the stage and supplicants would line up to be prayed for by the couple. Another common way healing was organized included pastors and their wives locking hands above their heads to create a "tunnel," through which individuals would run. Some would collapse in the tunnel, while others would become energized, only to run through again. Participating in these myriad forms of healing, however, required practice.

## LEARNING TO HEAL

> We call upon your authority so that you can help us. Your works, God, we need your holy anointing, have mercy on our team through the *mana* of your Holy Spirit this morning.
>
> —Hana

Each morning, the diabetes clinic began with a prayer. As the clinic filled with patients who would be seen on a first-come, first-serve basis, Mele asked an elder, usually a man, to lead the group in prayer. Elders would come to the front of the waiting area, an open-air room, enclosed with security bars, with rows of wooden benches for patients, as the clinic assistant keyed popular Christian hymns. After a few weeks, I was surprised to hear a common thread in Pentecostal prayers, one that was similar to the healing team prayer featured above.[6] They invoked God's mana to flow through doctors and medicines, saying things like, "God, love us and help the doctors with their duties so the mana of your blessings comes to them. Let them have understanding for their duties as we come wanting to get some help" or "We remember that your healing mana will be upon [the doctors and nurses] through the medicine they have prepared." Similarly, each morning, my adopted father would say a prayer over the medications he took for his high blood pressure: "Father, bless these tablets, let your mana make this medicine flow through my body." These kinds of prayers suggested that biomedicine—and its practitioners—were only effective because of God's power. By channeling God's mana through these health professionals, and their medications, Pentecostals incorporated biomedical tools into Christian healing efforts. Biomedicine was only a manifestation of God's desire for his people to be healed, revealing God's agency through the effects of pharmaceuticals. Doctors, nurses, and medicines were mere agents of God's power. Converts, however, had to learn how to "receive" healing by learning to see God as the source of healing, health, and health behavior change, something healers hoped to teach through their ministry.

At the hospital, the healing team gathered in the parking lot before entering the acute ward to pray. The ministry leader, Hana, would often pray over the team, asking God "for the mana of [His] spirit," to which the team would respond, "yes, Jesus." Her demeanor was serious as she said, "Our teacher, please come to open our mouths and let our lips speak, open our hearts so we can deliver your Word inside our dear country, Samoa. Let your mana be with all of us in the hospital to open the ears of your country to your Word." With this, Hana reminded the healers that they were effective because they were agents of God. They were not powerful healers themselves, but God, who literally put words in their mouths, made them effective. God also "opened the ears" of the sick so they could "receive" healing. Another afternoon, Hana prayed, "God, Father, open our hearts to listen to your word, the word of life. We call you this hour, let the mana of your blood Jesus clean us from our heads to our toes. Clean our hearts to listen. Your Word flows the mana to them. Father, you have the authority." These kinds of prayers instructed the women in a fundamental lesson that they would also teach: their successes were really God's successes. They could call upon the "blood of Jesus" to do the work of healing, but they were merely agents of His power, deferring their own individual talents.

When the healers worked with sick persons, their prayers always foregrounded God's agency. One woman who was suffering from an eye condition caused by unmanaged diabetes cried as one of the healers prayed over her: "You know everything from the head to the toe. Father we call you, the mana of your blood to reach our sister. My father, we call you. Nothing is impossible for you. We have the authority and the mana with us to destroy this sickness. We stand and believe in the authority and mana you gave us to destroy the sugar." These kinds of prayers suggested that there was nothing God could not do, making the supplicant responsible for their faith and indirectly their healing. When healers instructed that God was the source of healing, their task became focused on helping the supplicant develop their faith so that God's work could manifest, teaching new converts that faith was about *becoming*, an ongoing process of development.

In other instances, healers taught those they healed that they became sick because they were distant from God. One afternoon, Leti—a tall woman, with long gray hair tied in a low bun—and I approached a woman, named Tina, who was in her fifties, lying on her bed with her daughter beside her. Her legs were swollen, and it seemed to me they were twice their normal size, which I would learn later was a symptom of kidney failure. Tina knew Leti, and shared with her how being married to a matai, who was also a deacon in a mainline church, was causing her stress. Her legs had begun to swell a few weeks earlier, at which time she consulted with a *taulesea* (traditional healer). As they continued to swell, and eventually itch, she went to the hospital, where doctors told her that these were symptoms of unmanaged diabetes. After listening to her story, Leti calmly and softly explained that the team was in the hospital to complement the work of the doctors; while they healed the body, the team worked to heal the spirit. Leti explained why Tina's healing had not worked thus far, saying, "What is happening is because we can get lost inside the church." When the body is used for the "world of the flesh," it is susceptible to disease—through stress, eating, and competition, which the women felt was encouraged by mainstream churches. If you put the body to the work of eternal life, and abstain from selfish consumption, health returns. Tina's daughter hovered, as the three women cried and held hands.

Leti suggested that Tina was stressed and angry, and sick as a result, because she was distant from God. This distance was compounded because, even though she was active in church leadership, she did not feel she had a relationship with God. As a result, sickness could only be partially healed by the medicine she was being given in the hospital; spiritual healing was also required, which would allow her to change stressful relationships. The implication was that through her work in church leadership, she had become wrapped up in the competition and face-saving activities of church participation, not faith-based concerns of eternal life. Being born again promised her a way to be close with God and ways to avoid the temptations of the "flesh," like competition and appetite. In turn, salvation created the possibility for physical healing that would result from gradual spiritual transformation. Leti guided Tina through a healing prayer, which started with a salvation prayer and was followed by Leti "laying hands" on Tina. While the salvation prayer followed typical fashion—proclaiming Jesus Christ as Lord and Savior—Leti also prompted her to begin healing prayers by claiming, "I stand and believe in the authority and the power you gave us to destroy my sugar with your power." With her salvation prayer complete, Leti began the healing work. The woman trembled and whispered to herself, "I am a sinner." Leti laid hands on her legs, massaged her feet, and prayed over the affected areas. Leti commanded the "spirit of anger" and diabetes to leave her body. As Leti laid hands, she spoke to the foot and explained she knew God was inside of the leg. She said she knew this woman would change her anger and eating. Leti delivered the "spirit of anger" and diabetes, ensuring the woman that strength in her heart would be renewed. As Tina wept, Leti returned to her bedside and whispered diet advice—stay away from fatty food, buy juices from the supermarket, eat papaya. They said their good-byes and Leti hugged Tina's daughter. Leti embedded a healing prayer into the salvation prayer, and in doing so linked healing with Christian salvation. The two prayers became co-constitutive, with healing dependent on the completion of a salvation prayer. By reducing anger, eating fresh fruits and vegetables, and avoiding fatty food, Leti advised Tina on managing the body and relationships in a newly sacred fashion.

In other instances, healers taught people that by turning to God for comfort in times of suffering, healing could occur. Samaria, another member of the team, was particularly clear in her focus on comfort. Still wet from the sideways rain pulsing outside the hospital doors, one afternoon she sat down next to a middle-aged man whose foot was elevated and bandaged, fluids still seeping through. She gestured to his foot while stroking his hand and asked him why he was in the hospital—infected sores and numbness in his feet. "What a pity," she said. The team was in the hospital to work with the doctors and nurses, she explained.

The medical staff were good at providing "physical treatment to the body," but her team was there to "bring the miracle of Jesus." She asked him about his church—he was Methodist—and then assured him she didn't come to his bedside to bring "any religion or church" but instead to help him heal. "That is our message for you, brother, there is no one else who can give you healing and strength, only Jesus can." By being born again, Samaria promised him, "Those who believe in Him will be given the power of God so that they may heal." At this point, Samaria asked if he wanted to "accept Jesus." He agreed. "Close your eyes," she said, and "repeat after me":

> Jesus, Our Lord and Savior
> We fellowship in your goodness today
> Now we come before you
> We profess and declare with our hearts and mouths
> Our hearts believe
> We say to you Jesus
> Do come
> Do come and reign in our hearts
> Lord and Savior I believe
> Your blood is enough
> That flowed upon the cross
> That cleansed and washed my sins
> We call upon you at this hour
> Do come, and lead in my life
> So that you are the Lord, to save my life
> I accept you, please accept me
> Because I believe, and I have faith
> Only you are the Truth, the Way, and the Life. Praise You. Amen.
> Hallelujah, Lord. Yes, our Father, hear our prayers in this hour.

The man had neuropathy from unmanaged diabetes, and because he could not feel his feet, some sores had gone undetected and became infected as a result. After reciting this prayer, Samaria counseled the man to wash his feet regularly, to always wear shoes that covered his feet (not flip-flops), and to stop working in the plantation if he had children to take care of it—all of these changes would help keep his feet safe. She reminded him that God never gave people more than they could handle, but if he ever felt burdened, he should turn to God. Now that he was born again and had "the freedom to make the right choices," he needed to now "choose wisely" in his everyday life—to eat differently, to pay attention to his body, to wash and inspect his feet each evening. These changes won't be easy, she told him, but "take your burden, take your pain to Him, and He will give you peace. You only have to believe in God." Then she prayed for his healing: "Father, we are only vessels working for you. All healing is yours and that is why we call upon you. Your touch is needed upon him. Give your peace to his heart. Lift his pain. Dear Lord, let his skin grow back, the skin, the flesh. Father, you made us all in your image. Heal the body of this man as you had made him. This is our prayer, Father. In your Holy name, Jesus, Amen and Amen."

By starting with salvation and then reciting healing prayers, healers taught those who were newly converted that one depended on the other. Through this kind of medical evangelism, new converts learned that they needed to first turn to God for his healing power as a way of changing their health and health practices. Their own will alone was not enough; they needed God's power. These healers modeled deferred agency in their prayers by focusing on God's healing power that becomes available to people only when a person is born again. However, this was not an automatic process. When someone was born again, their infected skin did not automatically return to a healthful state. The believer needed to turn to God every day—seeking His healing power—"to receive."

## EMBEDDED NARRATIVES

Cluny and La'avasa Macpherson write that health and well-being means "accepting a Samoan view of the world and living by those customs, *o le aganu'u samoa* [Samoan culture], which support it. Conversely, the rejection of the worldview, and the customs, which underpin it, can lead to the imbalance, which results in illness" (Macpherson and Macpherson 1990, 157). Cardiometabolic disorders require shifting attention to the very fundamentals of health—food and body size, in particular—that often felt like challenges to Samoan culture. By embedding one's illness narrative into a conversion narrative, those living with cardiometabolic disorders could talk about health changes as a reflection of religious change while avoiding implicit critiques of fa'asamoa. Ordinarily, in everyday life in Samoa, talking about individual intentions, desires, and motivations is discouraged (Shore 1982; Mageo 1998; Anae 2016). Samoans, writes Alessandro Duranti (1992), are often more concerned with the repercussions of their actions than the intentions behind actions. By extension, talking about one's intentions and motivations or individual subjective experiences of suffering, for example, is typically subsumed by expressions of identities based on age, gender, rank, or office. Pentecostal conversion narratives mediate the tension between the cultural imperative to downplay individual desires, motivations, or suffering, and a Christian imperative to develop an individual, direct, and deeply personal relationship with God (Keane 1997a; Keane 2007; Bauman 1984; Robbins 2001; Shoaps 2002; Harding 2000).

Embedded narratives foregrounded the difficulties of adopting a new orientation to health and self-care by contextualizing difficulties in health as a reflection of spiritual difficulties. Narratives about self-care for cardiometabolic disorders often focused on the difficulties of paying diligent attention to diet, physical activity, and medication, which was not always feasible in this and other socio-economic contexts (Becker, Gates, and Newsome 2004; Clarke and Bennett 2013; Guell 2012; Seligman et al. 2015). For example, among Russian Jewish émigrés in the United States, "the prioritization of caring for the younger generations over themselves, their view of food as a vital necessity rather than an object of choice or desire" made biomedical self-care difficult, despite the fact they "acknowledge[d] the necessity of self-control in the abstract" (Borovoy and Hine 2008, 6). In other cases, narratives express barriers to food access or healthcare services (Carney 2015a; 2015b).

In the Samoa islands, scholars often report that the family is a source of stress and support. In particular, in relation to diet, there is a great deal of pressure to eat during regular family gatherings (Elstad et al. 2008; Rosen, DePue, and McGarvey 2008). Making changes to diet is difficult because families often share a single meal, while becoming more physically active often draws unwanted attention to the self. For example, one woman explained that when she exercised it raised suspicions about her fidelity. She said, people would snicker, raising an eyebrow as she walked by: "Why does she want to be thin?" The implication here was that concern with weight, and actively trying to lose weight, indicated a concern for appearance tied to sexual attractiveness. To lose weight, then, was to draw attention to oneself. Therefore, even physical activity could be interpreted as a self-serving action, one that publicly demonstrated how an individual was using time and money toward individualized self-improvement, which was thought to be at the expense of broader family well-being. Embedded narratives helped to make sense of the "human dramas surrounding illness" arising from individual struggles to make healthcare choices that impacted others (Mattingly and Garro 2000, 8).

Narrative analysis is now a common approach in the anthropology of diabetes because it provides a counter to medical, epidemiological, and genetic statistics often invoked in the study of cardiometabolic disorders (McCullough and Hardin 2013; Yates-Doerr 2013, 2015). "Statistics generalize," Carolyn Smith-Morris writes; in contrast, narratives "elaborate" (2006, 24). Narratives, sometimes called "lay discourses," are not "impoverished biomedical accounts," but are efforts to make sense of illness experience (Garro and Lang 1993, 294; Poss and Jezewski 2002; Becker et al. 1998; Naemiratch and Manderson 2006; Canaway and Manderson 2013; Lang 1989). Diabetes narrative analysis has shown how those living with cardiometabolic disorders are agents in managing their conditions, often despite steep experiences of marginalization and inequality. For example, Emily Mendenhall (2012) found a complex web of social stressors among Mexican immigrant women in the United States that often revealed a lifetime of chronic stress. By linking social suffering with disease causality, these women used diabetes as an idiom of distress (Mendenhall et al. 2010). Linda Garro's (1995) work with Ojibway people living with cardiometabolic disorders shows how stories about illness experience communicate disruptions to local lifeways due to European contact. Despite studies like these, local knowledge about diabetes, even though it influences healthcare choices, is often eschewed by biomedical practitioners (Schoenberg and Drew 2002).

Embedded narratives about conversion and diagnosis provided narrators a socially valued way to talk about the experience of making immediate changes to one's life around diet, physical activity, and consumption of tobacco and alcohol by picturing God as the agent of change, something shared across geographic contexts in conversion narratives. Pentecostals often maintain a language ideology foregrounding the power of language where "words come to create the very reality which they purport to describe" (Coleman 2000, 131). This language ideology reflects a "tight coupling of intention and meaning that is grounded in the postulation of a speaker who has both an ability and an inclination to tell the truth" (Robbins 2001, 905). When people become born again, they recite a brief prayer, whereby they proclaim a belief in Jesus Christ and make a commitment to dedicate their hearts and lives to him. This prayer is evidence of conversion and a means to transform the self. Saying words like, "I accept you, please accept me because I believe, and I have faith only you are the Truth, the Way, and the Life," changes the person from "unsaved" to "saved." In turn, the narratives that emerge about such events are "intended to create a spiritual crisis by calling to the fore one's desperate and lost condition, which one may have been totally unaware of" (Hill 1985, 26, quoted in Harding 1987, 170). Conversion narratives often unfold following "classic Protestant themes: hoping for personal guidance during a period of uncertainty; being led to an answer by seemingly coincidental and everyday but highly meaningful events; the translation of such events into a narrative that is repeated to others" (Coleman 2000, 18; Stromberg 1993). These narratives also celebrate and ritualize rupture with past lives as a way of foregrounding how change is derived by internalizing "the Word, the spirit, of God . . . when a person accepts Christ" (Harding 1987, 174; see also Meyer 1998; Engelke 2004). I draw attention to these kinds of common patterns to show how conventions of narrating spiritual crisis and rupture helped those newly diagnosed with cardiometabolic disorders to articulate their illness experiences.

Illness and conversion narratives are flexible genres providing a way of talking about individual transformation, foregrounding a "before" and "after" (Becker 1994). While chronic conditions disorder individual biographies (Becker 1997; Strauss 1984; Kleinman 1988), Pentecostal conversion narratives foreground rupture with past lives, representing "the process of becoming Christian as one of radical change" (Robbins 2007, 11). Ultimately, both types of narrative foreground disruption to the normal life course as a way to "make sense" of those events (Lang 1989:305). Based on narratives like Kika's, I show how the everyday disruptions to life that chronic illness often brings are addressed through the shifting of religious identity. By narrating illness experience through discussions of religious conversion, narrators strengthened their religious identities and foregrounded God's agency in creating change to their everyday lives, which they ultimately represented as the source of their ability to change their health behaviors. Religiously motivated change was a socially encouraged way of making changes to one's life because these changes suggest submission and obedience to God's will (Hardin 2016b). Embedding one kind of story about conversion, with conventions guiding the foregrounding of an individual relationship with God, into another kind of story about illness, where the convention is to minimize individual suffering, provides discursive tools for valorizing health behavior changes. In the examples I explore, embedded narratives demonstrate a performative confluence—conversion transformed health experience while talk about illness transformed religious identity.

Lua: "I thought I knew everything, I had everything under MY control." "Father's help" was the first explanation that Lua, a woman in her early thirties, offered when I asked her why she participated, nearly five days a week, in the popular Polynesian version of Zumba offered in Apia. A Pentecostal woman, who had "lost a lot of weight" through the help of God, founded these Zumba classes as an expression of her Christian "calling." After class, Lua and I met at a café, where we drank coffee and ate omelets as she explained how she felt she had changed her health. When Lua was diagnosed with diabetes, she was "feeling really sick." She was tired, she lost her hair, she had headaches, and she was "really grumpy." Moving from physical symptoms to cause, Lua noted that "one of the things that causes [diabetes] is stress." She reflected back saying, "In hindsight now, I look at it and I believe at that time, my lifestyle was really stressful." Even though she felt she was "having such a good time" and "partying," she realized after conversion that she was in "a destructive relationship," and that this was causing her a lot of stress.

By emphasizing the past stressfulness of her life and before conversion as a time in need of change, Lua represented her current "lifestyle" as different. She said, "I can say that now because my life, even though it's not, it's not totally as stress free as I'd like, it's so much lighter now than before." Lua would often talk about how, after she converted, she felt "lighter," metaphorically serving as evidence of better health. I asked her what had changed to make her feel "light." Before she converted, she said, "I thought I knew what I was doing. I thought I knew everything. I had everything under MY control. I thought I could change anything, I can change people, I control everything, that I was the queen of the universe." This "control" extended to personal relationships and the risks associated with "partying"—in this case, alcohol consumption, lack of sleep and exercise, and little attention to her diet. Born again, Lua realized, "I'm not [in control] and everything I was doing was just causing my body so much stress. Because I thought I can do all these things but no I can't. My poor body was just saying to me, 'Lua I don't think you can do that.'"

Lua felt this inner voice was God speaking directly to her through her body, which speaks to the health-giving properties of prayer that anthropologists are beginning to investigate (Luhrmann 2013; Corwin 2012, 2014). One of these properties is coming to know God as a loving interlocutor, one who provides support when needed. Coming to know God as a loving father, ultimately in control, meant Lua felt she needed to submit to God as a way of achieving health. This narrative is a "performance of submission," which elsewhere in the world is also seen as an "essential element of health" (Pitaloka and Hsieh 2015, 1155). Lua recognized her relationships and even her own body as out of her control, which helped her to see that there was "more out there that [was] out of [her] control." Once she realized this, she came "to know He promised healing" for mind, body, and spirit, once "you realize Father is in control." Realizing God was the agent of healing helped Lua make the changes she had struggled to make before she was born again.

Lua started visiting doctors, changing her eating habits, walking in the afternoons, and taking medication, although for weeks after she still felt sick. She vividly remembered this time as when she "hit rock bottom" and converted. "All I did," she said, was recognize the limitations of her own "strength" and "abilities as a human being." Realizing this, she said, made a "light go off," indicating that she needed to ask God for help. She cried, fell on her knees, and said, "Lord just help me." Immediately, she felt "peace of mind." Her eyes welled with tears as she said, "What a relief." For the first time in months, she felt she could sleep without worry, and from then on, everything seemed to work out in her favor. Foregrounding her ability to resist social demands as a form of deferred agency, she said, "I didn't do anything like what I used to do. Run around, do all these things." This running around "doing all the things" indexed prioritizing social demands of family and church above her own faith and health. Before converting, Lua was very active in her church, and as the youngest daughter of ten children, she was expected to take care of her aging parents, cooking dinners, cleaning the house, and watching her nieces and nephews when they returned from school. After converting, Lua didn't change her commitments to her family explicitly, but she did begin to prioritize her own Bible study group and Zumba classes, in turn lessening her daily commitments to church and family by virtue of opting to spend her time and money elsewhere. Lua was changing many things in her life, but she felt her conversion was the event that "changed everything."

Talking about her conversion helped Lua construct her story about learning to adapt to living with diabetes. Embedding her conversion story into her illness narrative encouraged her to connect struggles with these health changes with solutions provided by God, resulting from being born again. Just as Kika noted that "all" she did was walk on the seawall, Lua's transformative event was simple. She "submitted" by prostrating, crying, and asking God for help. God did the rest. Changing her health was easy after that, she felt, which was evidence of God's agency, not her own changes. Lua credited the event of her "yielding" to God as providing her the strength to go to Zumba, to eat differently, and to take her medications. Lua also used the metaphor of "lightness" to explain her health, which collapsed the distinction between embodied and social suffering. Her new experience of lightness derived from her relationship with God, which helped her change other relationships—she lessened her commitments to her mainline church, she stopped socializing with "unsaved" friends. Finally, Lua began to socialize with new networks of similarly aged Pentecostal women—going for coffee after Zumba or attending revival services in Apia.

Losa: "Changing my church cut the stress." When I asked Losa, a mother of five in her early fifties, if she had ever been diagnosed with a cardiometabolic disorder, she told me the story of her husband's sudden death. She learned her husband had diabetes, high blood pressure, heart disease, and kidney problems—"all of them," she said—when he was dying in the hospital. Losa was also diagnosed with hypertension and diabetes at this time (it was common for family members of patients to be tested when visiting the hospital). Losa thought the source of her husband's illness was stress related to family obligations, including cash contributions to church and ritual events. This cash poverty made him, and his family, eat "all the wrong foods." Even though he wanted to eat "more vegetables, more healthy food," the family did not purchase vegetables because money was prioritized for social networks. Losa described cash poverty, stress, and diet as interrelated causes.

At the hospital, one of Losa's friends invited a pastor from her Pentecostal church to visit with them, and they were born again. She said, "That is where I found salvation, the healing of that man, although he still died. It was not only the physical healing, but to me, it was the saving of his soul. He passed away but it started from there. He died, but he was saved." When Losa said, "it started from there," she referred to her conversion shifting the course of her life. Losa quickly switched back to discussing her husband's mainline church, saying, "My mind was heavy. I didn't feel free in that church." Giving to the church and family was a particularly heavy burden for Losa because, when her husband died, she had no way to earn money—her husband was a farmer who had sold produce at the market every day. Without his labor, Losa had no money. Losa's discussion of her "heavy mind" and lack of "freedom" was a reflection of this vulnerability.

Losa said that "everything changed" when her husband was born again, although she felt her high blood pressure acutely after his death—she often felt her "toto [blood] go up" when she felt "anger in [her] heart because of [his] family." Shortly after her husband's death, Losa began attending a Pentecostal church in the urban area, taking the bus for over an hour to attend this new church each Sunday. Over the course of a few months, Losa became an active church member, attending prayer groups and volunteering to work with the "healing team" in the hospital. Within a year, she was living on church land as a caretaker.

When Losa began attending the new church, this "cut the stress," and, like Lua, this made her feel "lighter." Now, Losa felt her high blood pressure was "good" because she did not feel the same stress. She didn't visit the doctor or take medication because she knew "Father healed [her]" because she "felt peace."

Just as Lua foregrounded conversion as *the* event that enabled her social life to change, Losa felt her husband's and her own conversion created her health as a proxy of her faith. Pragmatically, by embedding her story about conversion within her story about diagnosis, Losa was able to narrate how she made difficult changes to her life—withdrawing from demanding relationships with her in-laws as well as changing her church and residence. The metaphor of heaviness also collapsed the distinction between social and embodied suffering, allowing Losa to connect her stress with her cardiometabolic disorders. By focusing on her religious change, Losa was able to morally validate other changes in her life as a reflection of God's will.

Natia: "Jesus stopped the cigarette first." Natia's brother initiated her conversion and healing. When he converted, he changed churches, and as a result, the family stopped communicating with him. Despite living on a small island, Natia avoided contact with her brother for about five years, until he texted her to tell her that his daughter was in the hospital with *ma'i fatu* (heart disease). Iterating a common Pentecostal idiom, he felt this was because the family was "not of one heart;" it was divided because he changed churches. As a result, Natia's brother felt the only way to heal his daughter was to "unite" the family. Uniting the family, however, meant converting each member, so he called, texted, and visited family members, inviting them to his church, "just to listen."

As with the other examples, problems derived from family discord grounded Natia's conversion narrative. Visiting her niece in the hospital, and seeing how sick she was, Natia was encouraged to join her brother at church. "That was when my life was turned around," she said. Indexing the importance of the changed worship styles, Natia said she knew something changed when the praise and worship team sang. In her mainline church, she often sang, but "didn't feel anything. But this time when this church sang, the words of the song sank in my heart and I cried." This "different feeling" was the first thing she felt changed, and then the sermon seemed to be "Jesus speaking to [her] heart." Natia connected this personal, spontaneous, and intimate connection with God as a kind of discovery moment, where she began to connect sin, sickness, and her family suffering. She said, "I felt sorry for Jesus. There was a lot wrong in my life. I said to myself, 'He did not sin, but it was my sin that He was hung on the cross.' That day, God turned my heart around. There was a deep repentance in me. I humbled myself in front of God and through Jesus my life was saved from the depth of sin where I was." When the pastor announced an altar call for those who were "not saved," Natia walked to the front of the church and recited a salvation prayer. She remembered praying, "May God be kind and remove the poison in my heart. And bring His peace. To bring His peace and heal my heart." Natia prayed for her own heart, where sin associated with anger at her family's discord introduced "poison in [her] heart" and her niece's ma'i fatu.

When I asked her to explain how being born again could heal this "poison," she explained that "the reason [to be born again] is to return the heart to where it was, how it was given to you." In other words, all are born in a perfect Godly condition, but relationships and life circumstances often introduce sickness. When she was born again, Natia knew "God will take the heart to the condition he made it in body. It goes through the same process as God made it." To be born again was to refurnish the body with health, simultaneously healing physical illness and emotional suffering—often referred to as restoring the Kingdom of God on earth.

Conversion transformed Natia's relationships as she reunited with her brother, leading some of her other siblings to also convert. This change, Natia felt, also transformed her health. Natia connected her high blood pressure with anger, saying "anger in my heart was making me sick before that day." She remembered feeling her "blood going up," making her feel weak and dizzy before she was born again. Foregrounding God's direct role in her changing health behaviors, she said, "Jesus stopped the cigarette first." Natia had smoked for most of her life and struggled with quitting, but after being born again, she threw away her cigarettes and never went back. She did not take credit for this change; Jesus was the agent of change. After conversion, Natia also began to see a doctor about her high blood pressure, while also eating more vegetables and less fatty meat, and taking her medications every day. Despite these changes—social, affective, and medical—Natia credited her lack of anger and related newfound health to being born again.

As with the others, Natia highlighted God's agency in making changes to her health. She also foregrounded how changing her experience of church helped to create healing as she blended physiological suffering (derived from her smoking and lack of medications) with social suffering (derived from the discord in her family) as the cause of her sickness. Heart disease was thus a metaphor and a disease category, collapsing social, biological, and spiritual causes.

Embedded narratives foregrounded how conversion enabled these women to make changes to their lives that they felt impacted their health. Most strikingly, these narratives highlighted a convergence of diagnosis and conversion that, when narrated, elevated conversion over other simultaneous changes—like seeing the doctor, becoming physically active, or reducing stress—as the reason why the women felt healthy. Embedded narratives confirm that religion can play a role in how those living with cardiometabolic disorders interpret the meaning of their illness.[7] Whether food is pictured as a gift from God, or health is represented as being in God's care, scholars acknowledge how those living with cardiometabolic disorders draw from myriad religious resources to create well-being (Baglar 2013). However, looking to instances where God, church, or religion was invoked does more than assign meaning to the experience of suffering. Embedding stories of diagnosis and struggles to change health behaviors into a story about religious change frames health problems as religious problems, and thereby represents God as the source of health and behavior change.

These narratives pragmatically situated health in relation to the social context of suffering and faith as means to create change. In this way, these narratives demonstrate, as Mattingly and Garro observe, what "might not otherwise be recognized" (2000, 5). Specifically, conversion narratives encouraged newly born-again people to foreground suffering in ways that contrasted Samoan conventions around avoiding talk about individual suffering. By foregrounding God as the agent of change, this convergence created possibilities for those living with cardiometabolic disorders to talk about their everyday struggles to make changes to their health. Learning to adapt to a life disrupted by chronic illness, for many Pentecostal Samoans, was learning to narrate one's life as a "believer."

These kinds of embedded narratives show how those living with cardiometabolic disorders navigate multiple social pressures and healing choices simultaneously through the language of religious change. When Lua ceded "control," because God, not she, was the agent, she was able to change her relationships that she felt were the source of her sickness. When Losa left her family church, which she felt was the source of her husband's and her own sickness, she changed her networks by following the lead of the Holy Spirit. Natia, most clearly, refused to take credit for smoking cessation; Jesus was the agent. These examples together show the diverse ways that religious change provided support for health change and, in particular, illustrate how ceding one's agency in favor of God's agency was essential for these participants to change health behaviors. In other words, by converting, these women were able to make changes to their practices without risking criticism from friends and family. Being born again could be criticized by friends and family, and it often was, but conversion still provided a clear pathway for change in ways that changing one's health practices alone was not recognized or valued as an endeavor.

## FAITH IN WELL-BEING

To "control" cardiometabolic disorders, individuals must adopt health as a priority—an object of "personal effort, political attention, and consumer dollars" (Crawford 1980, 365). Viewed through the lens of Pentecostal Christianity, however, health became a measure of God's will and an object of His attention. As a result, healing cardiometabolic disorders involved learning to pray. It was learning to "let the Holy Spirit drive." It was letting God be the agent of behavior change. It was changing one's relationships to reflect one's new religious commitments. It was treating the body as a temple that God created. While maintaining health suggested concerns with weight, diet, and exercise, healing suggested a relationship with God that would make changes to weight, diet, and exercise possible because it was God's will. Healing was a process focused on learning to be close to God, to depend on Him, and to see health as consequence of Christian well-being.

Some Pentecostal Samoans used religious practice to negotiate their identities associated with chronic illness, by shifting self-blame generated from biomedical risk discourses to self-responsibility for religious practice. Learning to see God as the source of healing, and then embedding stories of illness into conversion narratives, helped those living with cardiometabolic disorders reformulate their identities in ways that facilitated some with health behavior change in socially valued ways. Healing, including the rituals of healing and the narratives generated from those experiences, transformed the resolution of sickness into an expression of religious commitment. Based on these arguments, in the following, I reflect on some of the consequences such findings have on medical anthropology approaches to chronic illness.

First, I suggest that medical anthropologists look to embedded narratives as a way of understanding how those living with cardiometabolic disorders navigate multiple social pressures and healing choices simultaneously. Looking to embeddedness "captures the relation of a narrative to surrounding discourse and social activity" and provides insights into how people living with cardiometabolic disorders transform illness experience into religious idioms for changing behavior (Ochs 2004, 282). New religious identities provide a socially valued mode of behavior change, while behavior change for health reasons is more difficult to sustain. This narrative convergence creates a normative way to talk about health problems as religious problems. In many contexts where religiosity is highly valued, by adopting a new religious identity, narrators can often create pathways for changing their health behaviors and sometimes move away from environments that constrained health.

Second, embedded narratives show how "historically informed genres," in this case, conversion narratives, help narrators make sense of their illness (Ochs 2004, 276). Examining how illness and conversion narrative genres interact is a way to understand how those living with cardiometabolic disorders call forth the resonances between Christian and biomedical ways of healing (Finkler 1994; Hardin 2016a; Klassen 2001a; Klassen 2001b; Klassen 2011). Instead of contrasting biomedicine and Christian healing, my interlocutors brought together these ways of healing to position self-care as religious practice. By telling stories about conversion during a medical event, narrators came to understand biomedical notions of risks (e.g., stress, diet, physical activity) as reflections of deficiencies in their religious lives. In this process, changing religious practice became a logical solution to the problem of cardiometabolic risk where diet, exercise, and pharmaceutical intake became problems to be managed with spiritual strength.

The narratives I highlight foregrounded relationships as risky to health, creating environments where individuals could not manage their cardiometabolic disorders optimally. Embedding shows how risk is locally understood within context, and, in turn, shows how everyday health behaviors become meaningful within a Christian framework of social action. Risk changes form from individually oriented risk (eat differently, exercise more, see the doctor regularly) to a moral choice (treat your body as a temple, let Jesus change your health, use money on your health). In turn, some of the social difficulties associated with changing diet, physical activity, and primary care are mitigated when interpreted through a Christian lens. Embedding narratives builds on the institutional pathways created once a person converts, as they are encouraged to meet with peers and church leaders to help orient their minds, bodies, and relationships differently to God. This combination of social support derived from what Pentecostals call fellowship, with the subjective transformations derived from new prayer and fasting practices, created social pathways that helped those living with cardiometabolic disorders attain well-being (see also Klaits 2010).

Directives like "eat more vegetables," for example, were interpreted through a series of questions about faith, encouraging believers to question the social impediments that stood in the way of achieving health as a manifestation of God's will. Who will be cooking? Who will buy the vegetables? Who will work the plantation? Who will prepare the taro? Healing, as a set of practices and ideas, provided believers with ways to connect these social questions with health consequences through a framework of God's support. This framing does not focus on institutional or structural constraints on food access, but does bring into focus that macro-level changes have impacted micro-level interactions.

As I sat in offices of the missionary school of Glory House, I asked one faletua about her efforts to heal her diabetes. She had to do her part, she felt, "so God could do His part." Despite struggling with her weight and diet, the faletua knew she had to deal with her "flesh" so that "the will of God can be established for me. When we do our part, then He will do His part." These fleshy desires include everything from appetite to being overly concerned with others' evaluations. Managing the flesh was therefore a way to cultivate closeness with God and positioned the responsibility to manage health as a responsibility to God. Health in this and the other examples is derived from God's power, but individuals had to manage themselves to bring that divine health into being. Striving toward Christian well-being over health created possibilities for change in how one oriented toward health as a priority and worked toward achieving health. These notions of Christian well-being encouraged converts to see health as social and divine accomplishment, in which care for health became an expression of faith.

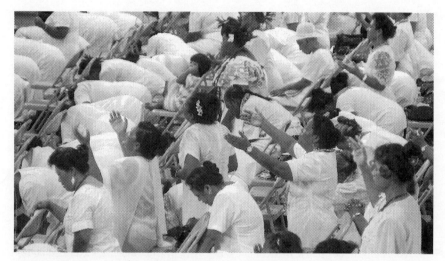

FIGURE 11 Every woman has at least one white puletasi. They are essential for some, each week, for Sunday services, and for others, for special services. On mother's day, each married woman (whether she had children or not) wore a white puletasi at Glory House. On this day, mothers were celebrated as the sermon focused on the role of women in the Bible, foregrounding particularly faithful women. Though the service was meant to show love and honor to mothers, mothers did a great deal of work to orchestrate the service. They performed songs or dances that they had rehearsed, for weeks or even months, to perform in front of the entire congregation. They performed in their cell groups, small prayer groups that comprised the larger congregation, as they met weekly for services.

# 7 · SUPPORT SYNERGIES

> Friendship ... is enjoyed proportionably as it is desired; and only grows up,
> is nourished and improved by enjoyment, as being of itself spiritual, and the
> soul growing still more refined by practice.
>
> —Michel de Montaigne (1891, 226)

Health, I have argued, is more than a set of biomedical metrics designed to measure the body—glucose levels, pounds, blood pressure. Health and its practices are embedded in the lifeworlds of individuals, which is one reason Kleinman calls for attention to local moral worlds, that is, for ethnographic accounts that show what is at stake in daily life for our interlocutors (1995, 45). Attention to lived values is an important counterweight to the "value judgments, hierarchies, and blind assumptions" that accompany a term like "health" (Metzl and Kirkland 2010, 1–2). Health is both "a desired state" and "a prescribed state and an ideological position" (Metzl and Kirkland 2010, 1–2). As a result, statements like "cut the salt" or "don't eat any fatty foods" suggest that a person who does not abide by those axioms is a bad person, one out of control (Greenhalgh and Carney 2014; Brewis et al. 2016). In contrast, and explicitly working to expand how scholars write about health, Emily Yates-Doerr and Megan Carney write about the kitchen as a site for care, calling for an "expanded vocabulary for health that recognizes health care treatment strategies that do not target solely the human body, but also social, political, and environmental afflictions" (2016, 305). I found that women created twinned social and divine support, which they mobilized over multiple forms of media, from texting to prayer to preaching, as forms of care that addressed individual health—as in an individual's "control" of their cardiometabolic disorders—and community wellness, through their evangelism as a means of creating God's Kingdom on Earth. These kinds of support bolster one another, revealing the ways that health is created through gendered friendships.

One afternoon in May, I arrived a few minutes before our regularly scheduled meeting time, before members of the prayer group at Glory House met to prepare for their ministry work in the hospital. I pulled up a chair in the office space that served on Sundays as the worship space for the English-speaking congregation and waited for the other women to filter in. Mother's Day upon us, the women chatted about the upcoming preparations for the celebratory Sunday service. When Hana, the ministry leader, joined, the meeting shifted in formality. She asked the women if they had read the Bible selection assigned last week: the story of Elisha raising the Shunammite's son, Book of Kings, which the women were to preach about on the church radio station later that afternoon. They reviewed the story for me. The prophet Elisha had promised a Shunammite woman a baby. Unexpectedly, after the baby had grown into a child, he died. When the child died, the mother returned to Elisha to ask for help. He came to see the dead child and returned the boy to life.

There are many potential lessons to be gleaned from this story, but the women focused on one dimension: the mother did not dwell in her grief or turn to her husband. After her child died, she had laid him down on the bed she kept in her house for the prophet Elisha, and said to her husband, "Please send me one of the young men and one of the donkeys, that I may run to the man of God and come back" (2 Kings 4:22). The woman had purpose and vision. Hana emphasized, "She walked away without saying anything to the husband." Later that afternoon, during the radio ministry, one of the women preached, "God made miracles. When the child died, the woman didn't even go to the father or take him to the hospital. When something is happening, you go directly to God. That's exactly where we should be, us mothers, if something happens inside our family. Don't worry, don't be afraid, be solid in your heart like the mother from Shunammite. She was a brave mother." I start with this Bible story and the women's interpretation to foreground how women cared for one another by generating synergistic support, both social and divine, through their fellowship. This is a kind of caring for health by creating an environment where women could reflect on their relationships and the ways those relationships impacted their well-being.

Writing of women's Aglow Fellowship, an interdenominational organization of charismatic Christian worshippers, Griffith focuses on the "healing power and transformative potential of prayer" harnessed through women-only fellowship (1997, 19). For women participants of Aglow, transformation is possible only in relation to women's capacity to surrender or submit to God and His demands (scriptural and prophetic). She writes, "Through prayer, a woman who feels angry, despairing, or powerless in her everyday life may experience a sense of intimacy with God as her loving father, friend, and husband. Through prayer, she can perhaps feel that someone hears her cry and cares about her pain, and that he will not only comfort her but will heal her suffering and fill her with joy" (Griffith 1997, 19). Griffith's vivid description describes how experiences of God can provide women with a sense of support, something the Pentecostal women I knew helped each other to create. This support is integral to understanding why health and faith are linked in Samoa and elsewhere: it allowed women to expand the ways they envisioned themselves as agents.

## DEFINING SOCIAL SUPPORT

Definitions of social support often include instrumental and affective support (Dressler 1980), including knowledge that one is esteemed and part of a network (Cobb 1976). Social support also provides an environment to cultivate identity and self-presentation (Keck 1994) and is linked to greater feelings of control, lower perceptions of stress, and less depression (Berkman et al. 2000; Uchino 2004). Social support also has particularly gendered expressions, something scholars have recognized as inherent to women's involvement in Pentecostal churches (for an overview, see Robbins 2004b). While men maintain formal institutional positions in churches as pastors, for example, women tend to rise to positions of authority because they are thought to be more sensitive to the movement of the Holy Spirit and therefore "receive" more gifts, which "underwrite their work as lay preachers, healers, evangelists, and prophets whose voices are often heard in church and other public settings" (Robbins 2004b, 132). Institutionally, as was the case with Glory House, Pentecostal churches often create all-female ministries, services, or prayer groups. These spaces provide women with opportunities to "develop public leadership skills and are often the one place in patriarchal societies where women can forge new relations outside their kin networks without exposing themselves to charges of immorality" (Robbins 2004b, 133).

Scholars have predominantly focused on the paradox of patriarchy in Pentecostal churches where women are submissive to men, while also providing space for "women's autonomy and equality" (Smilde 1997, 343). These studies focus on women's relationships to men and the various ways that patriarchy is at times reproduced and other times challenged (Brusco 1995). Jennifer Cole (2012), for example, reflects on how Malagasy Pentecostal churches assuage gender suffering related to social exclusion by providing women with alternative forms of authority rather than transforming their relationships with husbands and children, which are often the source of said suffering. Among Pentecostals in Samoa, I found women related to one another as agents of care in a social and economic context that required reconfiguring what it meant to show support for individuals and families—from food to prayer.[1] These women's groups helped each other with the kinds of everyday dilemmas I've explored throughout this book: healing cardiometabolic disorders required more than changing diet, exercise, and pharmaceutical intake; it required social transformation at the individual, family, and community level. It also required reformulating a sense of individual health and bodily autonomy. Through their membership in these groups, women worked on their health indirectly, by helping each other gain spiritual authority through their relationship with God.

## THE WOMEN AND THEIR MEETINGS

Hours before they were scheduled to leave for their ministry work, six to ten women gathered each week in Hana's cramped office. Glory House maintained offices in downtown Apia in one of the few remaining wooden buildings in the city. The building needed to be painted but remained a bustling place where congregants and visitors sought guidance and healing. The offices were also the site of church operations, and the smells of "sausage sizzle" fundraisers often wafted through the air of the building. The lead pastor's office was nested within layers of air-conditioned offices, while the women's healing team met in Hana's office, a room adjacent to the front doors without air conditioning. This subtle distribution of space reflects gendered church hierarchies. The pastors who were known for healing each maintained an independent practice—supplicants sought out the pastors individually, and the men operated out of their offices. The women's team differed. Hana, a serious and keen sixty-something listener, was the only member of the team with an official role in the church. Hana would remember each person's pains, symptoms, and heartbreaks and check in each time she saw them, while eagerly discerning the symptoms' demonic causes. While Hana was the charismatic center of the group, in part because all of the members had a relationship with her before joining, and participation was by invitation only, more senior women mentored more junior women, allowing for a cascade of mentoring. In fact, the most senior of Hana's mentees, Louisa, would act as the leader of the group in Hana's absence. Through these mentoring relationships, women learned to share authority, albeit in hierarchical ways. While the women who participated in the healing team were known to the congregation as a group of prayer warriors, they were not recognized individually through an official title or fulfilling a role in the church. They sat together each Sunday during services and were the most vocal section of the hundreds of people in the gymnasium and worship space. During the worship section of the service, the preacher would quieten the congregation in order to create space for "special messages from the Holy Spirit" that were almost always the voices of these women. However, these were "translated," if spoken in tongues, by men. Participation on the healing team provided some with social recognition of their "giftedness." In what follows, I explore examples where social support and divine support became intertwined in these meetings.

## "MAY GOD BE FIRST IN YOUR LIFE AND MY LIFE"

While activities varied, the ministry group regularly read scripture together, comparing translations and sharing interpretations and often focused on women of the Bible. They would describe women of the Bible as thoughtful and honest about their feelings with God. These characteristics defined women as responsible because of their faithfulness. Reflecting on the many women of the Bible, Natia said, "God has given great and mighty things to these women in accordance to the measure of their faith. In the same manner, we have to have that kind of faith." The group activities were thus as much about healing others as enhancing their own faith, which would make them more effective healers. They compared themselves to women in the Bible, as well as other women in their church. Through this comparative work, they together constructed a notion of an ideal Christian woman, while also creating themselves in the likeness of this image through their ministry work.

One afternoon before official activities began, Hana mentioned a woman she noticed at church who praised a little too loud. She said, "You must ponder over this. I want to turn back and say, 'Look, don't hallelujah but open your ears. Better to sit and learn the meaning of the service. Whether you're faithful or not, stop saying hallelujah too loud. The ears hurt. Don't interrupt with all those hallelujahs but be open and let the message come.'" With this example, Hana raised the specter of authenticity: was this woman really intimately close with God or was she just praising for show? She used this example as an opportunity to talk about disconnections between outward appearances and inward health. "This is the lesson for us, we go to church but sometimes how we live is very different." But, she reminded the group, "We don't judge people, right? But we take a look at the example, which is in this person." This woman's example showed members of the group that "from the outside," everything can look great, "she comes to church and praises." But inside could be different; the woman could be "living with sin, which creates a weak spirit." Her struggle was the struggle that all of the women experienced: pride interferes with faith. Hana made clear that the signs of being a "strong believer" could indicate the opposite: prideful practice. When she posed the hypothetical, "we don't judge," she persuaded the women not to condemn the woman but to see her as someone in need of guidance, and more broadly as in need of their help. This example also reminded the group that each of them shared this vulnerability.

Hana's description of this overly eager woman took group members from focusing on the outward signs of faith to the inward effects of inauthentic faith: a weak spirit. A weak spirit is one that is susceptible to sickness made manifest by evil spirits: the spirits of religion, pride, jealousy, or fear. Etiologies, in this way, are woven into ideas about faith. Hana made this connection explicit when she explained that she knew this woman was also "very sick" with "all the different sicknesses, because remember, when you are sick your body is weak. She has high blood pressure, diabetes, because right, you are worried, you are discouraged." Hana used this example to relate to each woman at the meeting; she asked them to consider whether they might be sick but not know it. This is especially relevant to cardiometabolic disorders that may be asymptomatic. Just like faith, health may seem outwardly present; deeper inspection might reveal invisible sickness.

The spiritual etiologies I have explored throughout this book depend on these kinds of general examples that can be queued up quickly. While Hana began this conversation casually, she transformed an observation about a particular woman into an investigation of a type. She moved the mode of investigation from the other woman to all Christian women, to the self. This conversational learning guided women through evaluation of those who were in need of healing, even those who were asymptomatic, while weaving together self-evaluation with health responsibility. Just as these women examined particular women as exemplar or lacking in some way, they also learned to evaluate themselves. This self-evaluation often focused on the difficulties of practicing faith, as the example of the Shunammite woman made clear. "Putting God first" was challenging because of family obligations and expectations that the women be submissive to their husbands, fathers, and pastors. So in addition to evaluating self and other women, these women developed strategies for cultivating authority and agency, so they could prioritize their individual relationships with God.

Members of this group learned how to prioritize time *with* God through prayer and fasting and time *for* God through ministry work, so providing them with tools for making choices that placed their desire for a relationship with God over other obligations. They accomplished this in part by consistently reminding each other that, although it was difficult, they were undertaking a divinely guided ministry. Reminding the women that "God [should] be first in your life and my life," Hana began a prayer session by saying, "Do the true things of God, because [the Bible] says, let's seek first the Kingdom of God and His righteousness." The women needed to turn away from sin, away from their "old worlds" and instead "go to Him." Once the women were saved, they needed to change everything: "Forget everything that you wanted, your children, family, or your husband. Now it's time for your soul." She ended by asking them, "Do you make God first, every Tuesday, Wednesday, and Thursday?" This question encouraged the women to self-evaluate and to place their everyday worries aside on the days when they undertook their ministry work.

Building on the example of the woman who worshipped loudly, Hana encouraged the women to take their relationship-building efforts an additional step, beyond participating in church services and prayer meetings. She asked them to commit private and individual time with God: "We should have our time to spend by ourselves. In the presence of God, the way is to pray, through fasting. I want to ensure, we have the time, so we are on fire together. Thanks to God. Sometimes, when we get to a prayer meeting, we look to others for what we should do. We pray, we fast. We listen to find what is inside of God, we talk about it. It's good to get to these meetings, it's good to listen, but maybe it's better to do it yourself and you get there yourself too. Through opening your heart to the Holy Spirit, and allowing the Holy Spirit to make you grow." First, Hana connected individual time with God with the effectiveness of the group, when she said that she wanted the group to be "on fire together." Then Hana focused on individual time dedicated to God outside the commitments of church and ministry. Hana encouraged the women to find their own ways to connect with God—that is, to take an active role in their devotion that extended beyond listening to sermons passively. In a separate prayer meeting, one woman shared that she would sometimes sit in the closet to get away from her children in order to have a quiet, dark space to listen to God.

Preaching on the Glory House radio show was a particularly clear way that these women bolstered their authority despite their exclusion from church leadership; it was also the only opportunity for women to play a public role. While the time spent together before the radio ministry often focused on developing confidence and an authoritative stance, on-air time provided women with the occasion to practice that authority. Before the women were about to go on-air, Hana reminded them, "Here is where you show what's inside your heart. So praise God, you trust God, He can lead." While ultimate authority was derived from God, these women were authorized as speakers of divine truth in part because they worked to cultivate that voice.

Prayers were directed toward God, asking him to grant the supplicant with divine authority. These authorization requests, which often began prayers and preaching, acknowledged a divine source while imbuing the speaker with sanctioned speech. In other words, prayer transformed the women from acting as individuals to acting as agents of God. Hana interceded on behalf of the women before they went on-air: "We have come to you with nothing. We don't know anything. May your love help us. We pray for the Holy Spirit, the Word of wisdom. God, in order to bring the Word of wisdom, Word of understanding in order to make things easy for us to feel the guidance of the Holy Spirit. We ask for your Holy Spirit to be with us. Teach us first. Thanks for your Spirit in our hearts. We ask for the communication between us, one person to another in order for us to cover what we forgot, God. Show us." These requests were not inherently gendered. However, when spoken in the context of a women-centered ministry, these requests contributed to a gendered project of enhancing women's authority as preachers and healers. When Hana marked the speech to follow as divinely guided, the individual women could trust in that authorization and "show what's inside their hearts."

These kinds of prayers fostered women's abilities to develop their own voices and provided them with space to make social choices—about their time and other resources—that in turn fostered their abilities to create closeness with God. This cultivation of voice was essential to how women created their own sense of well-being, in part because they could support one another while also learning new ways to seek support.

## "LET YOU, LORD, MEET ALL THE NEEDS OF EACH PERSON"

Social support is generated when kin and other intimate persons provide advice and help during times of need. However, in Samoa, where the dominant cultural model of self and social action is oriented toward understanding the social location of the self and acute awareness of an individual's effects on relationships, self-expression in the form of egocentric statements about subjective experience is limited (Mageo 1989; Mageo 1998). Self-expression is always implicated by its potential to impact a web of social relationships, which makes asking for advice or help difficult.[2] Duranti, in his work on oratory in Samoa, notes that complex social interactions regularly occur without "apparent concern with people's subjective states" (1992, 44), yet Pentecostal Christian practice encourages deep awareness of individual subjective experience. Healers, in particular, but all congregants in general, faced the difficulty of bringing out the subjective states of others. This was evident in the weekly ministry meetings where women did not express individual "needs" to the group. However, through text messaging these women directly asked for help.

Given that these women traveled from different villages on Upolu, without these weekly meetings before ministry work, the women would not know much about the other group members. Weekly meetings, therefore, provided opportunities for women to check in with other members, providing each other social support by sharing information about other group members, and sometimes people from the larger congregation. When team members did not show up for work, other team members discussed what they knew, and when they learned about a member struggling, they would discuss ways to help. For example, when one team member had not shown up for ministry work or church for a few weeks, Hana asked what the team members knew. Some had heard she was sick, while others had heard she was moving to a faraway village. After weeks of absence, Louisa (the second most senior woman in the group who Hana had mentored since the early 1990s) visited the absent woman and reported back that her move was not a good one. She was living precariously in the "back house" of her daughter-in-law's house, alone.[3] They described the house: wood and without walls, which meant the family was cash poor and had not been able to renovate the home into the increasingly common construction of a concrete structure with walls and louvered windows. The team collected some money for her, and Louisa visited again with this cash gift, though the woman did not return for many months.

On another afternoon, as we sat tightly arranged around the perimeter of Hana's office, women clad in puletasi pressed against each another in small chairs; the group organized a gift for Natia because she was traveling to New Zealand for her brother's funeral. For a few weeks prior, Natia had not participated in the ministry, which the group thought reflected her inability to travel to town—she did not have bus fare. Eventually, Hana convinced Natia to return by arranging her trans-port. On the afternoon she returned, Hana welcomed us and then asked Louisa to speak. This was the first indicator that a formal gift was going to be presented, as Louisa acted as a tulaafale for Hana, who in allowing Louisa to speak for her stands in for a matai.[4] Louisa explained that Natia would be leaving for a month: "We will show our support through your prayer and my prayer, follow her with our prayer we give in front of our God." She continued to pray for Natia to have cour-age as she faced her unsaved family. Louisa then offered a thin stack of cash from the group as a "small something to show our love for [her] trip." The linguistic exchange between Hana, Louisa, and Natia followed the pattern of *lauga*, formal Samoan oratory, which tends to be performed in the context of the *fono*, the meetings of the political organization of matai. Louisa's speech mirrored the seven-part lauga pattern: introduction, kava, thanksgiving, mornings, sacred titles, agendas, and clearing the sky (the official end to the speech)—though without the kava (Duranti 1994, 89–100). These similarities suggest kinship among the group, a group not otherwise bound by the webs of reciprocity built up over generations but nonetheless supporting one another. Using the formalities of exchange helped the women to reinforce their shared support of Natia and solid-ify themselves as a group.

Louisa also went to great lengths to distinguish this gift from a typical exchange relationship; this gift was not for fa'alavelave. Louisa even compared this gift to a time when a gift was collected for a previous member who had gone to visit family; Hana stopped the group collection because the woman was not in financial need and her family was "saved." Natia's trip was different as she had to minister to an unsaved family and she was in obvious need. While Natia had fa'alavelave obliga-tions, the money was for Natia's personal needs because the group knew Natia did not work and was largely alienated from her family (and thus from resources) in the islands. It was possible, still, that Natia would travel to New Zealand and find herself unable to meet her fa'alavelave obligations. In that case, Natia might use the money for fa'alavelave obligations, but the women framed the gift as money to be used by Natia for her personal well-being and divine purpose.

While this weekly meeting generated social support through the knowledge that each member was cared for by their community of women, no woman explic-itly asked for help during the meetings. However, through text messages, the women directly asked for support. Texting, in fact, was the cheapest form of communication, as it required minimal cell phone credit and often there were promotions, making texts free in the late hours of the evening. Though differing in age, among young women in Tonga, "use of . . . mobile phones presented opportunities for social interaction that would otherwise be too risky to conduct face-to-face while trying to maintain the image of an obedient, innocent young woman" (Good 2012, 177). Mediated requests provided these women with oppor-tunities for expression of interior subjective experience while not violating normative expectations for limited expression of personal desires. Texting for social support is an "idiom of practice" that mediates conventions for speaking about interior, subjective experiences (see Gershon 2010, 6).

Direct prayer requests via text were an everyday occurrence. One afternoon, I arrived several hours early for our meeting and found Lupe, a woman in her late forties, sitting and reading her Bible outside of Hana's office. Lupe shared with me that she was arguing with her husband over whether to contribute to her husband's family fa'alavelave. Her husband, like her, was in missionary school, which meant they were both living off savings from their previous careers as accountants. Lupe said she was "prompted by the Holy Spirit," to her surprise, to reach out to a new member of the ministry team. "In the flesh," meaning her instinct, she said, was to turn to Hana when she had a problem, or in her words, "a need." But she listened instead to the Holy Spirit, to try a new direction, and reach out to a relative stranger who was new to the group. Days later, when Lupe, Hana, and the new member met before ministry work, they were warm and chatty in ways they had not been before. These texts provided information about problems that would not otherwise have been talked about during the weekly meetings. By texting for prayer support, Lupe ensured God would intervene. She also inadvertently opened up a line of communication that permitted her to talk to a stranger about her personal problems. Texting prayer requests thus doubly mobilized divine support and social support, by enriching the relationship between texter and texted, calling forth God while minimizing individual expressions of suffering. Texting was therefore a form of social action that mediated concerns with morally appropriate ways of asking for help (see also Andersen 2013).

This group of women was in constant text communication. Newly converted, Ferila would text more senior women about everything from Bible translations to advice on how to pray. Ferila would text when she had a particular problem, and other women, in turn, would mobilize their prayer networks by sending a group text to "uplift Ferila," providing others with details of her particular problem. "Uplifting" was a way to ask God to speak to Ferila about her specific problems, which spanned problems from managing communication with her estranged husband to managing her mother's expectations that Ferila contribute cash to her family church.

While the senior women intended to mobilize God's support for Ferila, the effect was to notify an emerging social network that Ferila was in need. This provided them with the knowledge of a problem and, in turn, the intimacy and authority to speak to Ferila about it. While Ferila would not have come directly to this emerging network, she received social support from other women as she encountered them at prayer meetings or church. Uplifting as a text practice was the socially recognized way of managing a new convert's transition to deeper intimacy with God. It was a kind of recognition that a relationship with God could only develop when the believer had the capacity, knowledge, and tools to develop that relationship. Uplifting was, therefore, a way to socialize a new believer into her own relationship with God, allowing her to directly communicate with God while also embedding her in the new community.

For Pentecostals, God was source. He solved problems, provided myriad forms of support, and was an intimate and loving companion. Yet, new believers needed to learn how to ask and seek His help. Asking for assistance in ways that brought to light individual suffering is challenging in Samoa as there are few culturally explicit ways of asking for support other than directly asking for resources from family members to support formal gift obligations. In order to ask God for help, they had to first express their concerns and suffering, which they did differently depending on the communicative mode. Texting support was distinct from conversations, which shaped ideologies around the appropriate expression of self. In this light, social support was twinned with the experience of God as a source of support who met needs.

## "DON'T LOSE YOURSELF WHEN YOU ARE FACED WITH THESE PROBLEMS"

Social support was generated through socialization practices where both mentors and mentees solidified their identities as Christian women. By this I mean that when more "mature" women testified or witnessed—that is, shared stories of how God changed their lives—to women they mentored, they both performatively created themselves as strong Christian women and pragmatically guided others on how to seek intimacy with God. Witnessing God's power was a common genre among Pentecostal Christians, and anthropologists have long been interested in exploring how language shapes religious experience (see Keane 1997b). Susan Harding asked in her now influential essay on the rhetoric of conversion, "How does the language and performance of fundamental Baptist witnessing convict and convert the unsaved listener?" (1987, 167). Years later, Robin Shoaps asked, "How are prayers and songs of praise and worship crafted to meet the spiritual needs and reflect the ideology and identity of the group?" (2002, 32). In this section, I ask: How is social support generated through testifying? How are social support and knowledge of God's support related through this process of story telling? Testifying about problems by talking about divine solutions impacted the identities of both speaker and listener in different ways. For the speaker, these accounts created a Christian subject who was knowledgeable and faithful while also someone who supported other Christians. In these groups, as women responded to one another, or spoke about their own experiences, they could be esteemed by those who were listening. Meanwhile, listeners were socialized into the genre of witnessing, while also instructed on *how to ask* God for support.

Lagi led a Bible study group in her home each week, where she was particularly explicit about using prayer as an instructive tool. One evening, she began with a prayer where she directly guided others present to "search your heart and ask the Lord to search your heart." Emphasizing self-evaluation, she encouraged everyone to be "present" in this time of devotion. After the initial devotion time, Lagi spoke more freely: "God wants you to taste that the Lord is good. Oh my gosh, what He can do! He can stop the rain. Have I told you that? If you ask, God can do that. The angels will do it. God sends angels to do His bidding and His bidding depends on your asking. You ask God and God sends His army to come and do everything you want. Why? 'Cause you're His child." Lagi witnessed something as common as rain ceasing to demonstrate divine reciprocity. She relayed that God would provide everything one asked for, as long as the person asked. This God had angels who would do His work and so help individual Christians. This form of evangelism was particularly effective because "the use of autobiography and self-objectification . . . illustrates the ideal of a personal relationship with God," which is "deployed as a mode of persuasive discourse" (Coleman 2000, 119). Lagi's narrative created an image of God that showed Him as an active interlocutor, a familiar God, one who would provide support upon request if asked.

Lagi described her own relationship with God as an ideal way to teach ministry members about God's omnipotent capacities. She continued with her story about asking God to make the rain stop at a Gospel contest where she was acting as a judge. She and a friend held hands, stood together, and prayed in "the natural" (i.e., speaking in Samoan) and in tongues. "We both went off in tongues and then it stopped. The rain stopped. The program started." While she was praying, she told us, she said, "oh no, devil, you don't," and she "started rebuking." She then spoke directly to God, saying, "Father, there's a host of believers right here, right now, who want to worship you, who want to tell people about your glory. We want to celebrate you tonight, Father." Lagi's testimony about what she said to God and how she engaged with another born-again woman, Tai, was both a discursive practice of Christian self-making and pragmatic instruction for new believers on how to pray *in situ*.

Lagi was purposeful in offering a mundane example, later explaining to me that she kept her examples "simple" and "manageable" to meet the "level of spiritual development" in the group. She told the group she was able to stop dogs from attacking her, saying "in the Name of Jesus, and they stop. They don't do a thing." She also prayed over her son when he was "run over by a pickup truck" and "nothing happened then." Lagi shared these examples explicitly in response to another member's concern that she couldn't find time to pray. Lagi insisted that it would be easy once she started practicing, saying, "So I'm way over to the other side, I cannot go back. Same for you [gesturing to her], same for you [pointing to Ferila], same for anyone who comes to the Lord." When she said "same as you," Lagi implicated the group members as already having benefited from a personal relationship with God. In this way, she encouraged them to see the good things in their lives as having come from God.

Lagi suggested that this protection would only increase as they developed a closer relationship with God. "So I think you can go as far as you want to go," she said, before explaining that sometimes she also "backslides," but she "knows when I'm getting dry" that all she needs to do is turn back to prayer. When she doesn't want to pray, she knew that she was "almost on empty because I get busy with things of this world." Lagi talked about her own struggles—balancing her commitment to prayer with other commitments as a wife, mother, and daughter. She connected to the group by highlighting what she saw as the "benefits" they had all already experienced from beginning their "walk with Christ." The examples she offered all highlighted how the women managed to make choices that were counter to typical expectations and obligations associated with gendered roles. "Satan is very smart in throwing a lot of obligations," she said. He wanted people to be "busy with things, family, the church, things for work." These obligations were relentless, "so your prayer life just starts diminishing." These obligations made people neglect their relationship with God, which ultimately made people feel "stressed, angry, harboring unforgiveness." This was the "time to go back to the Lord." She then told us that, when this happens, "you've got to make a decision, to set a certain time aside for Him, even if it's 15 minutes, keep that time with Him." She used herself as an example. "I know I get bitter when I steal God's time, when I use God's time for something else." But "when God is with you, He will remind you. He will say helloooooo. Do you see what's happening? So you correct yourself. Right there and then. Say, oh Father God, I'm so sorry." Lagi was transparent that she was struggling with the same issues that Ferila and her other friends faced. She modeled spiritual growth and commitment, while also pragmatically advising them how to be close to God, setting aside fifteen minutes a day, for example, to develop a "prayer life."

Lagi also acknowledged that the stress of family and church commitments detracted from spiritual development. Like Hana, she encouraged the group to devote time to their own personal development over that of family and social commitments. The prayer meeting provided a space for Lagi to minister and guide spiritually younger women into a mature relationship with God. Lagi would cook for the women—making egg curry over rice, soy sauce–baked chicken, or *sapa sui* (Samoan chop suey)—allowing the participants to escape the difficulties of their own households and enjoy the company of like-minded women while "working on themselves," as Lagi would describe in English.

In other cases, women shared stories as a way of testifying about the effectiveness of God to create their own identities, while these stories also enabled them to support each other. When one woman discussed a problem she was having with her mother-in-law, Natia shared how, after her husband died, she cared for her mother-in-law who was bedridden and very ill. Natia tended to her every need, even fishing in the early morning for her favorite foods and making sure the household always had rice. Despite this, her mother-in-law was "very childish" and angry all the time. This was before Natia was born again, but she was certain it opened her heart to salvation through her struggles, noting, "I knew exactly the goodness of God." She advised the new member, "When [your mother-in-law] screams at you, go and kiss her, go to her. Combine humbleness and forgiveness." Sharing instances of divine support encouraged these women to continue to seek God, and to listen to the Holy Spirit.

Another team member shared that she had laid hands on her niece, who had an allergic reaction to a bee sting. Her sister-in-law accused her of "doing magic." The women in the group responded empathically when Louisa was reminded of the scripture Luke 12:10, to which the group opened their Bibles: "And everyone who speaks a word against the Son of Man will be forgiven, but anyone who blasphemes against the Holy Spirit will not be forgiven." Louisa said that many people who were not saved lacked understanding of the work of the Holy Spirit, and she reassured her fellow ministry mates that healing power did not come from individuals but from the Holy Spirit. "The fool doesn't want to know but there is the Grace of God to forgive, because they don't understand," Louisa said. Just as Louisa had assured Natia that the team would pray for her while she was gone, the group assured those with uncertainty that it was difficult to evangelize and love, forgive, and live with family members who were not saved.

Another dimension of social support was preparing the team for the rejection they might face as they evangelized in the hospital and among family members. One afternoon when preparing to enter the hospital, Hana began by saying, "Going out there today is not easy, we can see the anger in people's eyes and (see) that they are not happy, we can tell they don't want us there." But God was with them, "watching us from above." She reassured them, as some worried they wouldn't know what to say, that "God will give you the message and the words to meet them and the words for your prayer so you can pray for their illness, pray for their strength, pray for their return so they can grow again." She told them not to be surprised if people don't want to talk, "just pray to God." If they were willing to talk, she encouraged them to make a joke, make the person to whom they were ministering laugh, "to make them interested and listen to you." She reminded them that they were "selected for His work" and sometimes this work was difficult. "Don't lose yourself when you are faced with these problems"; instead just keep trying to reach people because "God already knows our plan for today and He is with us."

These examples bring to light what I have been referring to as the twinning of social support and divine support, or, more precisely, the knowledge of the potential for God to be a supportive entity. Asking God for help, imagining Him as an active dialogue partner, though, required practice. Women guided each other through this practice. For those who were speakers in a group meeting, testifying to women in need of support contributed to their own development as mature Christian women. For listeners, each story provided an opportunity to pragmatically learn how to ask and respond to God and how to manage family and community relationships. In their dedicated meetings together, the women reminded each other of God's presence by supporting one another.

## SUPPORTING WELL-BEING BY CULTIVATING GOD'S AGENCY

These exclusively women-only spaces helped the participants come to see one another, and the women of the Bible, as figures of Christian faith. They were reminded that trouble, problems, and struggle were part of this path. "We all face trials and tribulations in our everyday walk, in our families, workplaces," Hana said. It was normal to feel like "giving up," but in these times, she said, "just fix your eyes on Him and His divine calling. He alone will bless you. It's all about Him." These women constantly reminded each other that though their path was a divinely led one, it was not an easy one. Authorizing these women to make God a priority in their lives allowed them a degree of agency over their time, space, and obligations while often downplaying their individual agency. Through friendship and fellowship, these women developed their relationships with God individually, and so intimacy with God was a social as well as an individual process. These friends created the space and time to train and orient individual women to a new Christian worldview while also enhancing their own relationship with God and human others as more mature women. In these ways, these women's groups generated social support—which I show here as a network that a person can turn to in a time of need for help or advice, as well as a network that provided affective and instrumental support. The mentorship model is even implied in the terminology used to describe those who are newly converted, as "baby Christians" received guidance from "spiritually mature" women to cultivate new ways of relating to nonkin others, while also teaching them to develop intimacy with God. These twinned processes allowed women to dedicate time and space to develop their own authority outside the confines of kin and beyond other community expectations.

These friendships though were not ordinary friendships because they were institutionally created and therefore provided organized forms of support, which helps to illuminate an intersection of factors that impact health and well-being. As I outlined earlier, on the one hand, scholars have shown that social support can positively impact health outcomes. On the other hand, scholars have shown prayer or religious participation impacts health outcomes positively. My argument is not that these friendships were more effective in mitigating health outcomes. Instead, I have purposely focused on the dimensions of women's groups that correspond with the ways Pentecostals describe the cause of cardiometabolic disorders, evident throughout this book. Many of the dimensions of social support that I analyze here are not explicitly "health" related, and that is precisely the point I want to make. These women cared for one another in ways that created well-being.

Spiritual etiologies drew from medicalized notions of food, fat, and fitness—they connected diet, exercise, and pharmaceuticals with health—but they also pointed to stress, depression, and anger as important spiritual causes of cardio-metabolic disorders. These affective causes were social—they were states of mind that came from being in difficult relationships. The work of these women's groups addressed these difficult social relationships as a means to create well-being and, potentially, good health. As spiritual etiologies point to stress, depression, and cash poverty, these relationships provided opportunities for women to cultivate individualized agency while also providing social and divine support. In this way, these two forms of support were intertwined through the gendered social organization of women.

Pentecostal practice generated support that provided methods to achieving wellness that biomedicine neglected—material needs like cash, knowledge of a loving and available God, or a reliable social network. Women's practices were not explicitly linked to healing cardiometabolic disorders or any other illness; instead, organized women's groups shaped the social context in which efficacious healing could take place. In other words, as these women developed intimacy with God and other women, they also molded the obligations and relationships they saw as causing suffering and sickness—their families, their communities. Together, healing practices and Pentecostal gendered social organization helped to generate the religious experience of well-being.

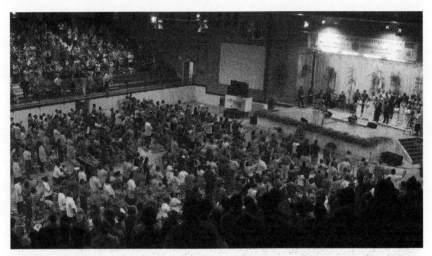

FIGURE 12 Twice a day on Sunday the national gymnasium filled with people from across Upolu. Buses crowd the grassy parking lot, some are church-branded buses—Kingdom Transport. There is a canteen, which mostly feeds hungry children to sustain them through the three-to-four hour services. Fizzy drinks, tuna sandwiches, instant noodles are offered. Adults don't eat. When I go to church with friends, we sit high up in the stadium tucked away from others we might know. When I attend with the healing team I sit in the front rows with only women. Even though there are over a thousand people present, sitting in these different places matters.

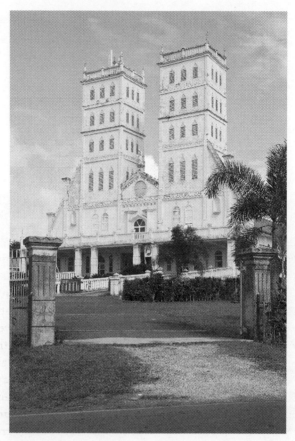

FIGURE 13 Every day I read the newspaper, retreating to the only air-conditioned room in the Nelson Memorial Public Library, where the Pacific Collection was held. In this small, dark room, there were four cramped tables, a copy machine, five years of the *Samoa Observer*, and a library attendant. I read the newspaper for stories about health and religion. What I found were stories about churches, pastors, and miracle foods or dangerous foods. The theological school graduations were always a multipage spread filled with photographs of pastors and their wives with lei stacked to their ears. Stories about lavish churches being built or tremendous fundraising efforts by church leadership. While I was there, a debate erupts in the "letters to the editor" section about whether Samoa should officially become a Christian state, and what constitutes a Christian. Years later the constitution changed to mark Samoa officially as a Christian nation. Food news usually consisted of two types of reporting—on the life-saving or health-restoring qualities of coconut, taro, or noni (*Morinda citrifolia*, a tree in the coffee family) and on the dangers of eating Chinese tinned fish, with photographs depicting contaminated tins with insects or rodents. The library attendant made photocopies of my dog-eared papers. After a few months, she asked about my research—unable to track the relationship between the kinds of stories I was clipping. She told me about her own church, and her own modest contribution to family meals. Her family called her Fa'i, which translates as banana. She didn't like it. The church pictured here is a Catholic Church, Our Lady of the Rosary, in Siusega. It is one of the churches that friends tell me to visit, for its beauty.

# 8 · INTEGRATING FAITH INTO HEALTHCARE PRACTICE

I began my research by following the expertise of people I met, from parking lot prayer meetings to emergency healing visits to hospitals, through food markets, pharmacies, and clinics. I did this ethnographically because, as João Biehl and Adriana Petryna write, "People on the ground recognize what's troubling them. And it is somewhere in the middle of their social lives that ethnographic work always begins" (2013, 18). In my fieldwork, I listened and observed how Pentecostals talked about suffering and worked to reduce it through their healing efforts. While the book started as a project about how Pentecostals managed chronic illness, what emerged over the writing was a broader critical reflection on how people understand health as a dynamic interface between God, community, and body. This approach, though, is not self-evident in healthcare infrastructures and cultures; it is an approach that Pentecostals worked to create. Living with families and creating enduring friendships showed me how people came to know their bodies through their relations to others. As blood pressure rose, it reminded people of the stress they felt from their families, yet when people felt at ease, they attributed this to God. This attribution of wellness to God is not unique to Samoa, but the examples I present here can speak to a broader process of socially mitigating the limitations of individual responsibility for so-called "lifestyle" diseases.

In *Faith and the Pursuit of Health,* I show how Christian healing created a sense of possibility among people living with cardiometabolic disorders. Healing helped them imagine change that was satisfying or at least intelligible. This focus on the ways that perceptions of what was possible—in health, relationships, and the community—was essential to healing because it distributed responsibility across many actors. Where biomedical and public health efforts constrained what seemed possible, attempting to convince people to eat healthy and exercise, Pentecostalism provided an organized set of scripts, practices, and rituals that expanded what seemed possible. For those who were born again during a time of illness, or those who reconnected with God after becoming sick, the pursuit and maintenance of health became an organizing feature of their lives because it became an expression of God's love. Aligning health with the duties of living a good Christian life made living a healthful life a moral life.

This stitching together of a healthful life as a Christian life became clear to me as I reconnected on Facebook with a pastor I came to know in Samoa. As we chatted, he told me he and his wife needed "to stay fit for God's work." I scrolled through his recent posts and saw that he had lost weight and was posting about this development. In one of his posts, he thanked his wife for supporting him, going to the gym with him, dieting with him, and sharing "her feelings with me." He also posted regularly to encourage his Facebook friends and family, and congregants, to "live healthy" because this is "God's will for His people." Whenever people judge you, he said, remember to be confident in yourself. Quoting Philippians 1:6, he wrote, "Being CONFIDENT of this, that he who began a good work in you will carry it unto completion until the day of Christ Jesus." On the one hand, this message communicates what it means to be a good Christian biocitizen—one who is fit for God. On the other hand, this message also shows how the pursuit and maintenance of health was more than a form of discipline. Weight loss, for this pastor, was possible because of support from his wife and God. His health was inevitable once he turned to God, and he found evidence of this in scripture. Health was a way to know about God's plan for him.

The role of agency is critical in this pastor's account, as well as in the examples I have presented throughout the book. While agency is a term that is widely debated in the social sciences, Laura Ahearn's definition is useful because of its breadth: "the socio-culturally mediated capacity to act" (2001, 112). Anthropologists have recognized that agency works differently for different people, varying in relation to cultural context (Ortner 2006; Mahmood 2005). In Samoa, there is a general suspicion of individual agency, and everyday life is guided by the hierarchical imperative to default to titled or other high-status people. Through prayer, healing, and narrative, however, the Pentecostals I met deferred their own agency by highlighting God's agency (see also Hardin 2016b). Other scholars have recognized this too; Julia Cassaniti writes that Christians in Thailand view personal agency as "enacted through engagement with an external Other" (2012, 309). Similarly, Hirokazu Miyazaki argues that Christian faith in Fiji emerges as the "capacity to place one's agency in abeyance" (2000, 32).

What is of critical importance in this book are the ways that this abeyance, or what I have talked about as deferring or de-emphasizing agency, is at the center of Pentecostal experiences of well-being. One could only be healthy or become healthy if God provided his *mana* to the medications that doctors prescribed, or if God provided the strength needed to purchase and eat healthy foods. To be healthy was less a matter of an individual's will than about bringing God's will into being. This cultivation process involved health techniques—like diet, exercise, and regularly presenting for primary care—but also broader efforts of striving for spiritual and economic prospering. As agents *of* God, the Pentecostals I knew were able to talk about, and sometimes actualize, changes in their relationships that were the sources of their day-to-day suffering. As an agent of God, Pentecostals could take chances and risk standing out against conventional norms around individual expressions of desires. In turn, they came to link social and economic suffering with cardiometabolic sickness, and developed ways to address health in an effort to create Godly well-being, thus bringing the Kingdom of God into the world.

When I started research in graduate school on the topic of diabetes and religion, I was excited to find a number of studies using churches as sites for interventions designed for Samoan populations (for some examples, see Aitaoto et al. 2007; Simmons 1998). In discussions with health workers, ministry officials, and other visiting researchers in Samoa, the church was often considered the lynchpin in creating sustainable social change. When I was doing fieldwork, government ministries enlisted pastors and churches to deliver programming—in the form of Jazzercise or educational campaigns. A common trope that health workers articulated was of a faletua sitting next to giant speakers blasting aerobics music as the congregants (or, more likely, the children of the congregation) danced on the church green. The importance of these kinds of public events rested less on the actual energy expenditure than on creating community awareness around cardiometabolic disorders. These kinds of publically visible community events are also sources of pride for churches as they are recognized as significant village institutions by virtue of their selection as a site for an intervention. Samoan public health has thus largely treated churches as cultural institutions from which to develop relationships with villagers, as they provide institutional inroads to villages as well as public spaces for organizing. However, conventional churches were usually the only churches selected as outreach sites. In selecting churches associated with village hierarchies, health becomes associated with politics. Bringing healthcare into villages is complicated because it matters through which relationship pathways that professionals enter villages. For instance, one physician shared with me that, during the national health fair, an effort to deliver primary care to villages across Samoa, a church had prepared meals for the visitors with the exact foods and portions she was planning to advise against. Yet, she had to eat. While entry into villages requires sponsorship from churches and matai, the accompanying rituals like a kava ceremony, speeches, or gift giving might cause village members to avoid the services, as there would be demands on them to provide food and gifts for their prestigious guests—doctors and government officials. From the perspective of people in the village, healthcare was expensive even when it was free.

Despite this, many health professionals remained deeply interested in how to work with what some saw as a strength of their Samoans patients and communities—their faith. This is where I think an ethnographic sensibility can be put to use in everyday life in clinics and public health offices. This sensibility is defined by radically listening—that is, listening to those living with cardiometabolic disorders about what resources they shore up in their efforts to cultivate well-being. Stacy Pigg describes something similar as the "practice of patient ethnographic 'sitting' as a means to understanding, as a form of critical reflexivity, and as a diagnostic of the politics of relevance" (2013, 127). I use the word radical to refer to the potentiality for listening to transform relationships on multiple levels—between health professionals and their patients, in churches and medical institutions.

Although this may seem obvious in a place like Samoa where I have described how everyday life is fashioned through Christianity, many health professionals I encountered felt they had to ignore issues of faith. Many of them were practicing Christians and did not want to "get in the way of an individual's relationship with God." Whatever people chose to do, one physician told me, "that's between them and God." Fasting is one particularly illustrative example of how a religious practice can have direct impacts on cardiometabolic health (Bloomer et al. 2011, 2012, 2015). Christians from across denominations fast in diverse ways as a form of prayer, communication with God, and sacrifice (see Hardin 2013). These practices differed widely from modest abstention from breakfast once a week to abstention from all meats for forty days—the so-called Daniel's Fast—to water only until the evening meal. Sometimes those who fasted also fasted their medications. These practices could have immediate consequences on glucose control, for example, yet healthcare providers preferred not to talk about religion. In these cases, patients were reprimanded for not maintaining "control" even while they were making efforts to maintain health. Radically listening could bring into the healthcare environment a focus on the social and subjective transformations possible when people draw from religious resources—like prayer or fellowship groups—while also recognizing the diverse ways that those living with cardiometabolic disorders try to care for their own health and the health of others. This suggestion—that something like listening can help to transform medical and public health practice—is not new to anthropologists nor to the Samoans I knew. Yet, it bears repeating because, as a practice, listening brings forward the perspectives on what matters in local contexts.

While research on cardiometabolic disorders demonstrates consistently the social foundations of the rise in these disorders globally—reflecting the intersections of poverty, gender, and geography, for instance—efforts to reduce these disorders still often target individuals and evaluate the success of such programming individually. Reframing local efforts to reduce cardiometabolic disorders might require thinking about what it means to operationalize a model of social care, mobilizing collective caring across institutional, cultural, and social boundaries (see Richards 2014; Taylor 2008). Public health in the context of Oceania might give leaders new tools for helping their faith communities, which would require dissolving reticence about working with Pentecostal churches—something that was evident in Samoa as working Pentecostal churches seemed to challenge political and social norms. Given that, as scholars and practitioners, we know that social environments shape experiences of well-being and suffering, we might better heed the ways that local communities, like many Samoans, recognize the value of religious frameworks for making individual and community changes in pragmatic ways—not only ritualistic and spectacular ways that are sometimes (and stereotypically) associated with Pentecostals.

Pentecostal discourses on cardiometabolic disorders reveal a religious version of the long-standing World Health Organization definition of health: "a state of complete physical, mental, and social well-being and not merely the absence of disease or infirmity" (WHO 2017). Health professionals—scholars, nurses, doctors, and health journalists—could learn to renarrate the stories of epidemiological change in similar ways that Pentecostals in Samoa do: from looking to prevent the emergence of cardiometabolic disorders to looking to the creation of spiritually sustaining communities. Shifting from a language of deficiency, deprivation, and reduction to a ministry of caring for all could mobilize more people in health practices.

# ACKNOWLEDGMENTS

There has never been a piece of writing that I have written and rewritten in my mind more often than these acknowledgments. When writing challenged me, I'd think forward to this moment of communicating my gratitude as a mindful retreat, savoring the process of tracking the social life of this book. I'll start with where I sit as I finally draft this section—at a writing retreat at Pacific University. Starting with where I sit now is a technique I learned with my students—looking through foggy windows as Oregon winter beats outside, tackling what feels like a momentous task—writing ethnography in their senior capstone projects. Yet as I wrote alongside them, and my colleagues at Pacific, a manuscript became this book. I am grateful for this community that has created a nourishing environment for writing.

The book's first life as a dissertation was supported by faculty, staff, and fellow students at Brandeis University. Richard Parmentier guided me through research by insisting I wait until fieldwork was complete to analyze and make conclusions. This trained patience is something I am still cultivating, making me grateful for the intellectual space that this kind of waiting produces. Sarah Lamb and Elizabeth Ferry provided endless feedback, support, and pragmatic advice from my first days of graduate school to this day. For others at Brandeis, including Janet McIntosh, Caitryn Lynch, Megan McCullough, Ellen Schattschneider, and Laurel Carpenter, thank you. My time at Brandeis has also brought me friendships I cherish, who have sustained me as I worked through graduate school into my first days teaching—Emily Canning, Casey Golomski, Anna Jayesane-Darr, Brianna Mills, Mrinalini Tankha, Nurzhan Sterbenz, Angela Stroupe, thank you. During graduate school, I also spent time at UCLA, where Alessandro Duranti and Jason Throop provided critical feedback as my fieldwork was just beginning to develop. There I also met Anna Corwin, whose friendship and intellectual affinity (and feedback on so much of my writing) I value deeply. During fieldwork, my friendship with Christina Kwauk sustained me. My life in Samoa has also been guided by Fepuleai Lesai Iona Mayer, Jackie Fa'asisila, Galumalemana Steven Percival, Maria Kerslake, and Silao Kasiano, fa'afetai. While in Samoa, I learned (and still learn) from Meleisea Leasiolagi Professor Malama Meleisea, and Penelope Schoeffel, as their depth of knowledge is a source I have come to greatly admire. Most recently, Alex Brewis and Amber Wutich have provided cherished mentorship, imparting much-needed models for living life as a woman scientist. To Lenore Manderson, I am especially grateful. Her belief in the project was rejuvenating, and her meticulous and skillful commentary and editing have greatly strengthened this book, and has changed how I think about writing.

Through the years, and countless conference papers and writing projects, I have had the great privilege of feedback from and conversation with Ping-Ann Addo, Eileen Andersen-Fye, Anne Becker, James Bielo, Leslie Butt, Megan Carney, Simon Coleman, Risa Cromer, Tom Csordas, Elizabeth Dunn, Hanna Garth, Ilana Gershon, Susan Greenhalgh, Deborah Gewertz, Courtney Handman, Nicola Hawley, Hillary Kaell, Jennifer Hirsch, Pamela Klassen, Stacy Langwick, Stephen McGarvey, Amy McLennan, Emily Mendenhall, Sally Merry, Kathy Oths, Nancy Pollock, Joel Robbins, Rochelle Rosen, Ryan Schram, Bradd Shore, Cindi SturtzSreetharan, Ty P. Kāwika Tengan, Matt Tomlinson, Sarah Trainer, Susanna Trnka, Catherine Trundle, Emily Wentzell, Paige West, Ian Whitmarsh, Fa'anofa Lisa Uperesa, and Emily Yates-Doerr. Chapters of this book were also presented at the National University of Samoa, Yale University, University of Washington, the University of Auckland, and Columbia University. Audience members, especially, Lesley Sharp, Adrienne Strong, J. C. Slayer, Julie Park, and Judith Huntsman, provided valuable feedback. To colleagues and friends met through dedication to ASAO, Mary Good, Tate Lefevre, Chelsea-Wenthworth, Marama Leigh Muru-Lanning, Alex Mawyer, Alex Golub, Albert Refiti and Melani Anae, it has been my great pleasure to think alongside of each of you in shaping the contours of Pacific Studies.

Writing is also the everyday work of sitting, sometimes with others, and sharing nascent work. For this companionship, I am grateful to Barbara Andersen, Annie Claus, Ram Natarajan, Moriah McSharry-McGrath, and Dawn Salgado for their continued "accountability." To colleagues at Pacific University, who helped me balance writing, research, and teaching, I am grateful to my department as well as the enduring presence of my mentors, Jules Boykoff and Rick Jobs. Over the years, this research has been supported by grants from Fulbright-Hays, the Firebird Foundation for Anthropological Research Grant, the Wenner Gren Foundation, and Pacific University. At Brandeis, several sources supported this work, including the Fannie and Simon Shamroth Endowed Fellowship and the Otto and Mynette Bresky Endowed Fellowship, the Mellon Foundation, the Department of Anthropology, the Department of Women's and Gender Studies, and the Graduate School of Arts and Sciences.

Fieldwork has been one of life's greatest privileges as I was welcomed into strangers' homes and churches. This willingness to teach a stranger, and tolerate her as she learned, was a generosity that was the norm not the exception in Samoa. I am deeply indebted to Leiloa Asaasa, Lua'ipou Kisa Faumuina, Dionne Fonoti, Jordanna Mareko, and Mele Mauala for their help navigating new relationships and providing much-needed feedback and context for many of the observations made in this book. Mafi Palepoi-Tulia, in particular, provided friendship, humor, and kindness, and much-needed space to think critically about the kinds of observations I was making day to day. I would have been lost without her. Agnes Kerslake, our connection always astounds me. Thank you for being my guide. I am also grateful to the leadership and staff at the Ministry of Health and the clinics that hosted me, providing support, information, and sage guidance on the complex health issues that face Samoa.

My deepest gratitude goes to the communities that brought me into their homes across Samoa. ʻO le tusi lenei o se meaalofa faʻatauvaʻa e ʻavea ma faʻamaumauga o le g āluega tāua tele a ʻilātou ʻuma ʻoloʻo nafa ma le tiute o le togafitiina ma le tausiina o gasegase, ʻo ʻilātou foʻi ia na tatalaina mai o lātou ōlaga iā te aʻu. Faʻafetai tele i le tou agāga ālolofa. ʻUa ʻavea lava le tou ālolofa e fai ma mea ʻua sui ai loʻu ōlaga. Apulu ma le ʻāiga, faʻafetai i lo ʻoutou ālolofa ma lo ʻoutou agalelei na ʻavea ai aʻu ʻo se tasi o tagata o lo tou ʻāiga i le taimi na ʻou moʻomia ai se ʻāiga. Agnes, sā ʻe taliaina aʻu, ʻo se tagata ʻese, i lou ʻāiga ma ʻavea ai aʻu ʻo se uso ma se uō iā te ʻoe. ʻO le tōmai ma le sosia na ʻe faʻasoaina mai ʻo se meaalofa tāua tele lea i loʻu ōlaga. Apulu, o lou poto ma lou onosaʻi lea ʻua tino mai ai lēnei tusi, ma ʻua ʻavea foʻi lea ma taʻiala i loʻu ōlaga. ʻUa ʻavea ʻoe ʻo se tamā iā te aʻu, ma ʻo se tūlaga lea e lagona ai loʻu faʻatauvaʻa ma loʻu maualalo. ʻOu te tuʻuina atu foʻi le faʻafetai faʻapitoa iā Apulu Puʻa Fonoti ma Aiono Lonise Apulu ma Ps. Faumuina Alofa Faumuina ma le faletua o Tafaoga Faumuina. Faʻafetai tele lava. I Ekālésia ʻuma ma alālafaga na tatalaina mai o ʻoutou faitotoʻa faʻatasi ai ma o ʻoutou loto iā te aʻu, FAʻAFETAI. ʻO sesē ma aleu o lenei suʻesuʻega, ʻo ā aʻu ia.

Finally, my family has buttressed my life as a fieldworker. For this, I am grateful to my parents, Peg and Mel, and my in-laws, Bob and Chris, for encouraging and supporting me as I traveled—and continue to travel—for long periods and insisted on writing through travel, holidays, and even the briefest of visits together. For my parents, I am particularly grateful for the curiosity you gave me, and general wonder with the world and its people. Finally, for Greg, your enduring companionship, humor, and inexhaustible support fill me with gratitude. I cherish our life together, now with George, as we make it our own every day.

# GLOSSARY

**ai:** eat

**alofa:** love/generosity

**fa'aaloalo:** respect

**fa'alavelave:** ritual exchange; anything that interferes with normal life and calls for special activity; accident; important occasion; trouble

**fa'asāmoa:** the Samoan way; Samoan culture

**fale:** house

**faletua:** pastor's wife

**fe'au:** chores

**fono:** political meetings of titled leaders/chiefs

**ie'faitaga:** men's formal lāvalava

**kokoraisa:** rice cooked in Samoan cocoa and coconut cream

**lapo'a:** big, fat; tino lapo'a is technical translation of obesity

**lāvalava:** cloth used like a sarong

**lotu fou:** new churches

**ma'i fatu:** heart disease

**ma'i suka, suka:** sugar sickness; diabetes; sugar

**malosi:** strong

**mana:** sacred power; power; God's grace

**matai:** titled political leaders, chief, general term refers to both ali'i (high chiefs) and tulafale (orators)

**meafai:** obligations to church or family

**pālagi:** European/white people

**pisūpo:** tinned corned beef

**puletasi:** Samoan women's clothing

**tālā:** Samoan currency

**taulasea:** traditional healer

**tautua:** service

**to'ona'i:** Sunday meal

**toto maualuga, toto:** high blood pressure; blood

**upu fa'aaloalo:** respect words

# NOTES

## CHAPTER 1    SALVATION AND METABOLISM

1. This research was conducted in Samoa, formerly Western Samoa. Samoa was the first Pacific Island to become independent in 1962. American Samoa, a group of islands adjacent to Samoa, is an unorganized and unincorporated territory of the United States.

2. I focus on the clustering of cardiometabolic disorders, as opposed to diabetes only, because people in Samoa often experienced many disorders at once and also treated each disorder generally in the same way (see Seeberg and Meinert 2015 and Manderson and Smith-Morris 2010 for a critique of the NCD framework).

3. EFKS is one of the three main congregations; the others are Methodist and Catholic.

4. To talk about the "fire of the Holy Spirit" indexed charismatic practices of glossolalia, the phenomenon of speaking in a foreign language through which the Holy Spirit communicates to the speaker or listeners, or prophecy, the ability to predict God's plans.

5. Typically, Christian demonology reveals culturally specific negative attributes of persons, but some are shared across global Pentecostalisms (Csordas 1994, 181–185). I found four categories of spirits most commonly referenced. The first category includes negative human attributes that are aligned with the Samoan hierarchical ethos and result from discontent with the status quo: pride, anger, jealously. The second category of spirits includes unforgiveness, anger, or bitterness, which result from particular events in one's life that are thought to cause physical illness and spiritual suffering. In this category were also the "spirit of the strong man" and "the spirit of Jezebel," which could be introduced through inappropriate sexual activity, usually, as a youth. The "spirit of the strong man" was explained to me as the spirit that enters a young girl as a result of inappropriate sexual contact with men, usually, through sexual abuse. The "spirit of Jezebel," on the other hand, was introduced by consensual sexual activity. Sex before marriage could also introduce the "spirit of lying." A third category of spirits was specifically related to faith and church institutions. The "spirit of unbelief" was, as it sounds, in someone who did not truly believe in God and referred to the devil's "stronghold" on a person's spirit. The "spirit of religion" indicated that one was captivated by religion and religious performance without a relationship with God. Finally, the fourth category of spirits included particular sicknesses: diabetes, high blood pressure, stroke, schizophrenia, cancer, or depression. Spirits of cancer or infirmity inhered in particular places in the body and required targeted healing (Csordas 1994, 196). For example, it was common to see healers speaking directly to body parts—a painful knee or a back—or to lay hands on cancerous areas of the body.

6. This focus on the interconnections between individual and collective salvation is similar to that which Robbins (2004a) found among Urapmin Pentecostals in Papua New Guinea. He argues that a dyad of sin and salvation mediate Urapmin tensions between individual and relational notions of what it means to be a person.

7. Pacific Islander bodies have also become synonymous with sport, including rugby and American football (Uperesa 2014; Uperesa and Mountjoy 2014; Kwauk 2014b; Besnier 2012; Tengan 2002; Tengan and Markham 2009). Micronesia, especially Nauru, has also become a place synonymous with obesity (see Zimmet, Arblaster, and Thoma 1978, 1990; Zimmet et al. 1990; Eason et al. 1987; Balkau et al. 1985).

**8.** See Harvey and Cook (2010), Polzer (2007), Polzer and Miles (2007), Doucet-Battle (2012, 2016), and Mitchem (2007, 2010) for explorations of the intersection of Christianity and diabetes management among African American communities. Another domain where there has been robust study of the intersection of illness and Christianity is the anthropology of reproduction and HIV/AIDs (Inhorn 2012; Dijk et al. 2014; Prince, Denis, and van Dijk 2009; Burchardt 2015; Golomski 2014, 2015a, 2015b; Smith 2004, 2014).

**9.** I use the term Oceania to refer to Polynesia, Micronesia, and Melanesia and emphasize the interconnectedness between islands and cultures, while also avoiding the reification of European categories of regions (Hau'ofa 1994; Tcherkezoff 2003; Clark 2003; Thomas et al. 1989; Jolly 2007). I also use the term Pacific Islands and the Pacific interchangeably, following the health science literature as needed.

**10.** I use the term spiritual to talk about the ways that believers conceptualize a relationship between the self, what Csordas calls "the sacred self," and God. I focus on spirit, following my interlocutors in how they divide a person into three parts—mind, body, spirit—to parse how they see the spirit as a mediating space between mind and body. This is similar to how Seligman defines self as the "intersection of the mind–body. It is an emergent product of both cognitive-discursive and embodied processes; in other words, processes at both levels are in constant feedback with one another in the creation and maintenance of self. Both are implicated in threats to and disruptions of self and in its repair" (2010, 298).

**11.** Despite the everyday entanglements of health and Christianity in Samoa, there has been little research at this intersection in Oceania (for work in Melanesia, see Eves 2010). In part, this is because the study of medicalization arose out of an interest in the apparent decline in religious authority where problems once deemed moral, social, or legal (e.g., alcoholism, drug addiction, and obesity) become medical. For example, starting in the latter part of the twentieth century, medical jurisdiction began to take a greater and greater role in regulating everyday life, showing how medicine is an agent of social control, "supplanting 'traditional' institutions of religion and law" (Lock and Nguyen 2010, 67; Zola 1972). In turn, when life course problems are translated into medical problems, conceptual and institutional frameworks for addressing those problems are also transformed, including "fundamentally transformed ideas about the body, health, and illness, not only among experts, but also among populations at large" (Lock and Nguyen 2010, 69). In eighteenth-century Europe, childbirth, for example, once the domain of midwives, became the domain of the medical profession, transforming with it ideas about female agency and passivity (Lock and Nguyen 2010, 48).

**12.** See Brewis (2011) for a discussion of the BMI classification system and Yates-Doerr (2013), McCullough and Hardin (2013), Trainer, Brewis, Hruschka, and Williams (2015), and Jutel (2006) for a discussion of the limitations of BMI as a measure.

**13.** The social life of Pentecostals has recently come to the fore of the anthropology of Christianity (Bialecki 2009; Handman 2015; Haynes 2013; Robbins 2009; Marshall 2009), which has largely focused on the cultivation of an authentic, spontaneous, and individual subject (Harding 1987; Shoaps 2002; Luhrmann 2012).

**14.** There is an emerging literature on Christian-based weight-loss programs (Griffith 2004; Gerber, Hill, and Manigault-Bryant 2015; Gerber 2012, 2015; Bacon 2015) and the role of the fat body in classical Western thought (Hill 2011). There is also a robust literature on muscular Christianity (Alter 2004; Kwauk 2006; Wilde 2004).

**15.** Pentecostals were concerned with three primary domains of mediation that articulated a broad critique of obligation: worship, interaction norms, and giving. First, the ritualized predictability of mainline services was deemed problematic because prescribed forms of worship inhibited developing an authentic relationship with Christ. Another focus of critique was directed at the respect protocols required for interacting with elders, pastors, and matai. I often heard critiques of the ways formal language was used in mainline churches, saying things like "the youth can't even understand the sermons because of the *upu* fa'aaloalo (respect words)." A final dimension of critique focused on the formal organization of gift giving thought to reflect "human laws, not the Bible way," which was thought to be tithing. In each of these critiques, Pentecostals focused on how the institutional organization of mainline churches inhibited individuals from developing an intimate and spontaneous relationship with God.

16. An extensive anthropological and public health literature documents the role of *susto* in diabetes etiologies among Mexican and Mexican immigrant communities (Hunt, Valenzuela, and Pugh 1998; Jezewski and Poss 2002; Loewe and Freeman 2000; Mendenhall et al. 2010; Mendenhall 2012; Poss and Jezewski 2002; Weller et al. 1999, 2008; Thomas et al. 2009). This *susto* etiology is a "series of economic, social, or relational factors that produce fright in participants and together 'cause' diabetes" (Mercado-Martinez and Ramos-Herrera 2002, 797).

17. I use the term "adopted" because of the primacy of kinship in Samoa as a mode of relating. I also followed the lead of my host family as Tanu introduced me as his daughter to people in the village and congregation. By stepping into the role of "adopted" daughter, my presence in the village made sense in a locally meaningful way.

18. Tanu's assumption reflects Mead's (1928a) observations that dance created spaces for Samoans to express individuality while cultivating skill at a very young age.

19. Tanu's narrative echoes what other anthropologists have found across the world: Pentecostal Christianity traffics in a deeply gendered ideology of personal change (Eriksen 2012, 2014; Robbins 2012). Scholars have focused on the ways that Pentecostalism assuages women's gendered suffering by offering them alternative sources of authority to challenge, manage, and cope with difficulties in their relationships with men (Cole 2012; Brusco 1995). Scholars are also increasingly turning to Christian efforts to shape masculinity (Klinken 2012, 2016; Bielo 2014).

20. Not surprisingly, Good describes a parallel between "fundamentalist Christians" and "a-religious scientists and policy makers" to unpack this problem of belief (1994, 7). He argues that these two types share a model of individual transformation where belief should change individual behavior as a way to bring about healing. The model suggests that if institutions educate about risk or false beliefs, individuals will take up new beliefs and, therefore, create new life, health, or salvation (Good 1994, 7). Scholars of Christianity, on the other hand, have argued the problem of belief rests in the assumption that there is a mirrored relationship between behavior and interior experience. Critical of this premise, Lindquist and Coleman have asked: "What is the relationship between belief and the ordering of existence? Is belief a necessarily individualized and internalized phenomenon? How do we understand the connections between belief and experience, whether the latter is constituted by ritual or by ordinary activity?" (2008, 4). Both belief paradigms suggest a rational individual subject who changes behavior based on knowledge.

21. Klassen also proposes four vectors of analysis that help to explain how "concepts of religion and spirituality help to establish the legitimacy and authority of specific approaches to healing" (2014, 69). These include "*historicity*, by which healing 'traditions' are cultivated; *supernaturalism*, by which the power of divinity is both imagined and channeled; *postbiomedical embodiment*, by which the authority of biomedicine is absorbed and sometimes challenged by those who are not medical experts; and *political economies*, by which access to diverse modes of healing, including biomedicine, is differentially allocated." I find postbiomedical embodiment and political economies particularly helpful ways to understand the cases from Samoa where this combined attention to the ways that the integration of biomedicine and faith healing is shaped by access; they bring to the fore of attention how healing is a practice of critique.

22. See Csordas (1994, 168–171) for a more in-depth discussion of the discernment of spirits.

## CHAPTER 2    ETHNOGRAPHY BETWEEN CHURCH AND CLINIC

1. For example, Congregational missions dominated missionary activity in Samoa, and there was an informal agreement between John Williams, the first missionary to arrive in Samoa, and the Methodist church (then the Wesleyan church) to focus their energies on different islands—Congregational in Samoa and Methodist in Tonga. However, as Tongan relatives traveled to Samoa, they shared the news of the Methodist church in Samoa, and shortly thereafter, matai invited the Methodist missionaries to Samoa as a way of creating distinctions between families.

2. For more on the diversity of healing traditions in Oceania, see Parsons (1985), Macpherson and Macpherson (1990), McGrath (1999), Marshall (2012a, 2012b), and Moyle (1974).

3. There are several Pentecostal churches local to Samoa, including Worship Center and Peace Chapel, as well as others that originate elsewhere, including the Church of the Nazarene, Rhema All Nations, and Open Brethren. From the census data it is apparent that membership in mainline churches is slowly declining, while membership in Pentecostal churches and other lotu fou—the Church of Jesus Christ of Latter-day Saints, Jehovah's Witnesses, Seventh-Day Adventists—is slowly increasing.

4. Cell groups were groups who regularly met for Bible study, usually lived in geographic proximity to one another, and acted as parachurches.

5. I use the term faletua throughout the book to highlight the importance of this role in Samoa, as there is a term specifically for the pastor's wife.

6. The great majority of land in Samoa is customary land; in other words, most land is tied to families and particular matai titles. Only 4 percent of land is freehold, which means it can be purchased; another 15 percent of land is government owned. This land was originally seized by the Germans but returned to the Samoan government upon independence (Macpherson and Macpherson 2009, 66).

7. At the time of long-term fieldwork, on Upolu, there were four clinics, and on Savai'i, there were three clinics, in addition to a referral-based hospital. There were several private practices, although these were more expensive. There was also a dialysis center and a diabetes clinic, both sites where I conducted fieldwork. At the time of writing this, a new hospital was being built with Chinese aid.

8. The primary care clinic is housed in the former hospital, which now stands adjacent to the new buildings.

9. No home glucose testing kits were available in Samoa at the time of long-term fieldwork, so patients could only have their glucose tested in medical facilities. People could of course purchase them overseas and travel with them, but they were not available for commercial distribution.

10. An abbreviated version of this chapter appeared in the Field Notes section of the *Cultural Anthropology* website as "Fat: Translation" (April 12, 2015; https://culanth.org/fieldsights/662 -fat-translation).

11. Definitions of "indigenous" are contentious, and "it is not a term with wide currency" in the Samoan islands (Uperesa 2010, 281). The term indigenous is "inherently situational, hybrid, syncretic, and articulated as it is grounded in genealogy and land" (Tengan 2005, 253; see also Diaz and Kauanui 2001).

12. This interpretation of Mead's work follows Freeman's claims; some have pointed out that he was led by the orthodoxy of male elders while Mead focused on the perspectives of girls (see Shankman 2009).

## CHAPTER 3    DISCERNING AMBIGUOUS RISKS

1. While this might seem to reflect an ethnoetiology about cardiometabolic disorders, the assignment of a spirit cause and the discerning of that spirit is a typical expression of Pentecostal healing.

2. For example, in 2002, 20.7 percent of the adult population worked full time (Samoan Bureau of Statistics 2012), which is highest in Apia, where 35 percent of the population worked for wages or salary (Samoan Bureau of Statistics 2012).

3. Many matai hold more than a single title (sometimes as many as twenty or thirty), and residence in the village where the title originates is not necessary. This diversification, commodification, and proliferation of titles can create tensions within villages and families (Yamamoto 1994; Tuimaleai'fano 2006). Families that once "spoke with one voice" in various political forums, including the fono, "are now beset with tensions that reflect competition between titleholders for power within families, or for the right to administer family land" (Macpherson and Macpherson 2009, 127).

4. For a history of fat in Euro-American contexts, see Stearns (2002) and Hill (2011).

5. Rubin and Joseph (2013) also argue that African American women in the United States are caught in the cross hairs of public health as both populations who exemplify "protective factors" against obesity and are high risk for obesity for the same reasons—fat neutrality or positivity.

6. These fat-positive attitudes have been linked to high rates of obesity (Brewis and McGarvey 2000), although scholars have found a downward shift in idealized body size from Samoa to American Samoa to the diaspora in New Zealand (Brewis, McGarvey, and Swinburn 1998; Brewis 2011; see also Becker 2004).

7. Besnier, writing of Tonga, suggests that the stillness of dignity contrasts with joking, clowning, and gesticulating, which is a form of a "histrionic hexis" that conjures "sexual undertones" by drawing attention to the body (2011, 218).

8. This is similar to how Yates-Doerr found that environmental concerns with pesticides often made it a healthier choice to opt for highly processed, high-sodium, and fat-dense foods over locally grown produce because of environmental concerns (2015, 32).

9. This reflects what has become the hegemonic approach to food in global health, nutritionism, the reduction of food value to nutritional components (Scrinis 2008).

## CHAPTER 4    FREEDOM AND HEALTH RESPONSIBILITY

1. Meafai means "things done." The word fai means "do," but here refers to cash, other forms of material wealth, and labor contributions, and mea again means "thing." Another commonly used word for meafai is saogamea, which can be broken down into its constitutive parts in order to best understand the meaning. Mea means "thing," and the prefix sao means "save." Thus saogamea is literally "things saved."

2. Similarly, Mageo describes how "egocentric" orientations are displaced by sociocentric orientations, writing that "personal thinking, feeling, and willing are not distinguished: one term encompasses all three events" (Mageo 1998, 10; 1989, 191–192; Gerber 1985).

3. In preparation for hemodialysis treatment, people need to undergo surgical procedures to create an access point to their bloodstream, called a vascular access. The access point allows the patient's blood to circulate within the dialysis machine.

4. Prayer warriors are soldiers "who fight on Christ's side in a spiritual war" (Luhrmann 2012, 155). Being known for "praying powerfully," as in American evangelicalism, "was distinctly good" (Luhrmann 2012, 155)

## CHAPTER 5     EMBODIED ANALYTICS

1. The RSA (Returned Servicemen Association) is a popular bar in Apia.

2. Portions of Chapter Five previously appeared in a different form in *Fat Studies: An Interdisciplinary Journal of Body Weight and Society* titled, "Fat Studies Christianity, Fat Talk, and Samoan Pastors: Rethinking the Fat-Positive-Fat Stigma Framework" (2015;4(2):178–196).

3. Mana is defined in Samoan as divine power or God's grace (Anae 1998; Schoeffel personal communication, November 2, 2015). The Samoan definition resonates with Hawaiian definitions of mana as "power originating from a spiritual source" (Silva 1997, 91) and the Māori notion of mana defined as "power, prestige, authority, control, 'psychic force,' spiritual power, charisma" (Salesa 2011, ix). Marshall, also writing of Hawai'i, suggests that mana is "more than a theory, mana is a relationship and a practice that in precolonial times was the source of health, vitality, and abundance, in which a thriving world was the co-creation of divinity, humanity, and nature: fractal and indivisible" (Marshall 2012a, 88). Most broadly, mana "is an indigenous ontology" (Marshall 2012b, 88; see also Kame'eleihiwa 1992; Shore 1989; Valeri 1985) and "a pan-Polynesian concept of divinely sanctioned power and efficacy" (Henderson 2010, 310). It is also spiritual power and prestige (Tengan, Ka'ili, and Fonoti 2010) and spiritual authority and sovereignty (Meleisea 1997, 469).

4. See Saguy (2013), Rothblum and Solovay (2009), LeBesco (2011), Greenhalgh (2015), Boero (2013), and McCullough and Hardin (2013); for more on the negative meanings of fat, see also Taylor (2015).

5. The link between gluttony and fatness, however, is not new. Exploring the ancient roots of this link, Hill finds "a pervasive and continuing strand of cultural thinking in the West that disparages overindulgence and privileges moderation and self-control" (2011, 2). Unlike today, however, Hill finds distinctions between being fat and being gluttonous where positive associations with fat persisted, thus showing the ways the meaning of fat and eating not only vary cross-culturally but also change over time.

6. Protestant Christianity has shaped largely secular ideologies of body size around weight loss, food restriction, and moderation in eating (Bacon 2015; Hesse-Biber 1997; Fessenden 2006; Pellegrini and Jakobsen 2008; Gerber, Hill, and Manigault-Bryant 2015).

7. An additional way Christianity was Samoanized was by incorporating the pastor/congregation relationship into the *feagaiga* (covenant of mutual respect). This covenant relationship is ideally one of complementarity—that is between those of "equivalent rank or position in parallel hierarchies" (Shore 1982) The pastor/congregation relationship ideally mirrors the brother/sister relationship where the "village is the brother who holds executive power and the pastor the sister who holds rights to consultation" (Macpherson and Macpherson 2009, 107; Tuimaleai'fano 2000, 172–173). This is parallel to the ways that, in mainline churches, the "pastor provides the congregation with moral guidance and 'the good word,' while the congregation in turn supplies the pastor with money, food, and a place to live" (Shore 1982, 206).

8. These annual gifts include the *fa'amati* and the *Me*. The *Me* is an offering for the national church to fund missionary work, capital investment for church construction, support of senior church members, and other national church funds. Amounts are suggested at the village level. The *fa'amati* is the annual gift designated for household improvements for the homes of pastors and their families.

9. At the time of writing (2017), this roughly converted to USD$29,000 to USD$56,000.

10. Part of the reason Telisa was vulnerable to Ioane's family demands was because she was a *nofotane*, which is a term that refers to a wife living with her husband's family. This is a difficult position to be in, as the wife is expected to care for the household, often a thankless job. In

fact, there is growing concern about the abuse and vulnerability that nofotane often face, leading many women's organizations to create awareness campaigns.

11. This indicates the devouring speed by which Lagi engaged with American Pentecostal Christianity, and in particular the theology of John Hagee and Joyce Meyers—both who converse in the concept of a counterfeit.

12. Globally, this end times framework highlights the differences between local traditions and perceived universal truths (Handman 2015; Robbins 2004a). For example, in Papua New Guinea, Robbins argues that millennialism is a way for Urapmin people to balance the demands of tradition with Christian demands of individualism. Urapmin strove to create a relational form of salvation, attempting to "save their church in a way that honors relationalism while skirting the demands of Christian individualism," which suggests that salvation is an individual experience (Robbins 2004a, 303). Lagi delicately navigated the value of individualism and relationalism when she focused on transforming Samoa and its leaders by working in a prayer group that "stands together." Lagi aimed to transform one institution (i.e., mainline churches, government) by working together with her fellow prayer intercessors, not by individual efforts. Certainly, her individual message from the Holy Spirit placed Lagi in a special position in this venture, but change could only be achieved by working together in unity.

13. Anthropologists are increasingly looking to how Pentecostals understand the importance of unity. Among Auhelawa speakers of Normanby Island, Papua New Guinea, Schram shows how they use an "ideology of 'one mind'—unity in purpose which is subjectively felt and outwardly expressed—to resolve how their collective worship related to individual belief" (2013, 30). See also Handman (2015) and Hardin (2016c).

14. At the time of writing, WST$100 converted to roughly USD$40.

15. Lagi's vision and her mentoring were a form of everyday millennialism, "which consists of a constant round of talk about the imminence of Jesus's return and the moral vigilance needed to make one ready for his arrival" (Robbins 2004a, 303). Robbins argues that millennial ideas "endeavor to devalue traditional living and laboring arrangements—and thus establish the claims of Christian morality as primary" (2004a, 303). In Lagi's example, the authority of leaders was devalued to establish the primacy of her peers as a source of authority. The pastor's body symbolically clarified differences in these forms of authority.

16. Traditionally, scholars have used the term performative to refer to the ways certain utterances transform identities (Austin 1962). For example, by saying, "I now pronounce you man and wife," a minister transforms individuals into their new roles as husband and wife.

## CHAPTER 6    WELL-BEING AND DEFERRED AGENCY

1. Portions of this chapter appear in a different form in the article "Embedded Narratives: Metabolic Disorders and Pentecostal Conversion in Samoa," which appeared in *Medical Anthropology Quarterly* 32(2): 22–41.

2. For more on the limitations of health metrics see Adams (2016) and Merry (2016). For more on analytic frameworks for distinguishing between health and well-being, see Izquierdo (2005) and Mathews and Izquierdo (2009).

3. For more on learning to live with diabetes, see Ferzacca (2000), Borovoy and Hine (2008), Warren et al. (2013), and Canaway and Manderson (2013).

4. Based on a randomized controlled trial, Luhrmann and Morgain (2012) show that prayer cultivates the inner senses, which in turn helps to create a loving-relationship with God and may contribute to good health: "Mental imagery grows sharper. Inner experience seems more significant to the person praying. Feelings and sensations grow more intense. The person

praying reports more unusual sensory experience and more unusual and more intense spiritual experience" (359). Corwin (2014) deploys linguistic analysis to find that, among elderly American nuns, prayers mitigate loneliness and chronic pain at the end of life.

5. A particularly well-studied intersection of religion and illness is that of cardiometabolic disorders and Christian practice among African Americans (Doucet-Battle 2012; Doucet-Battle 2016; Polzer and Miles 2007). For example, knowledge of God's role in illness management positively influences self-care for chronic illnesses among Christian African Americans (Harvey and Cook 2010). Even further, perceived spiritual care from a healthcare provider facilitated self-management of diabetes among African Americans (Polzer 2007).

6. I participated in and observed at a diabetes clinic where I audio and video recorded morning prayers. These prayers varied from brief prayers lasting a few minutes to prayers lasting up to twenty minutes. Prayers were always followed by a song. After the prayers, I would ask the supplicant his denomination and also others in the clinic in order to learn perceptions about prayer styles and formulas.

7. For articles that all draw from religious examples, see Poss and Jezewski (2002) Scheder (1988), Schoenberg and Drew (2002), Weaver and Hadley (2011), and Yates-Doerr (2012a).

## CHAPTER 7   SUPPORT SYNERGIES

1. Similarly, the HIV/AIDS epidemic in Botswana has shaped how Pentecostals love and care for those suffering with the disease, as "love and care for others ideally enable[s] them to prosper"—making these sentiments relational (Klaits 2010, 6).

2. Asking for material assistance to meet obligations among family members is quite common. In fact, at least among Samoan migrants, they practice a form of strategic ignorance about the resources of family members (Gershon 2000). In other words, Gershon explains, it is the "job of those receiving the appeal to establish the limits of the resources as strategically and inoffensively" as possible (2000, 84). This form of seeking reflects the fact that "Samoans are not so much concerned with knowing someone else's intentions as with the implications of the speaker's actions/words for the web of relationships in which his life is woven" (Duranti 1992, 42).

3. This assessment reflects the morality of spatial orientations in Samoa where the front of houses or villages is associated with positive dimensions of sociality, while the back is associated with evil spirits and backwardness (see Shore 1982). To say someone is from "the back" is to suggest they are backward as well.

4. Orators are lower-ranked titles, but are engaged in a reciprocal relation with their chiefs, exchanging their service to the chief, including speaking for him during fono, for protection and material support.

# REFERENCES

Adams, Vincanne. 2016. *Metrics: What Counts in Global Health*. Durham, NC: Duke University Press.

Addo, Ping Ann. 2013. *Creating a Nation with Cloth: Women, Wealth, and Tradition in the Tongan Diaspora*. New York, NY: Berghahn Books.

Ahdar, Rex Tauati. 2013. "Samoa and the Christian State Ideal." *International Journal for the Study of the Christian Church* 13(1): 59–72.

Ahearn, Laura M. 2001. "Language and Agency." *Annual Review of Anthropology* 30:109–139.

Aitaoto, Nia T., Kathryn L. Braun, Dang L. Ka'ohimanu, and Tugalei (lei) So'a. 2007. "Cultural Considerations in Developing Church Based Programs to Reduce Cancer Health Disparities among Samoans." *Ethnicity and Health* 12(4): 381–400.

Alexeyeff, Kalissa. 2009. *Dancing from the Heart: Movement, Gender, and Cook Islands Globalization*. Honolulu, HI: University of Hawaii Press.

Alexeyeff, Kalissa. 2013. "Transnational Anthropology: Pacific Perspectives on Migration, Culture and the Imaginary." *The Australian Journal of Anthropology* 24(3):338–344.

Alter, Joseph S. 2004. "Indian Clubs and Colonialism: Hindu Masculinity and Muscular Christianity." *Comparative Studies in Society and History* 46(3): 497–534.

American Diabetes Association. www.diabetes.org/in-my-community/awareness-programs /american-indian-programs/. Accessed April 27 2017.

American Diabetes Association. www.diabetes.org/living-with-diabetes/treatment-and-care /high-risk-populations/treatment-american-indians.html. Accessed December 27 2017.

Anae, Melani. 1998. "Fofoa i Vaoese: The Identity Journeys of New Zealand Born Samoans." Ph.D. Thesis. University of Auckland, New Zealand.

Anae, Melani. 2010. "Teu Le Va: Toward a Native Anthropology." *Pacific Studies* 33(2):222–240.

Anae, Melani. 2016. "Teu Le va: A Samoan Relational Ethic." *Knowledge Cultures* 4(3):117–130.

Andersen, Barbara. 2013. "Tricks, Lies, and Mobile Phones: 'Phone Friend' Stories in Papua New Guinea." *Culture, Theory and Critique* 54(3): 318–334.

Anderson-Fye, Eileen P. 2004. "A 'Coca-Cola' Shape: Cultural Change, Body Image, and Eating Disorders in San Andres, Belize." *Culture, Medicine, and Psychiatry* 28(4):561–595.

Anderson-Fye, Eileen P., and Alexandra Brewis, eds. 2017. *Fat Planet: Obesity, Culture, and Symbolic Body Capital*. Santa Fe, NM: School of American Research Press.

Anderson, Ian. 2013. "The Economic Costs of Non-Communicable Diseases in the Pacific Islands: A Rapid Stock Take of the Situation in Samoa, Tonga, and Vanuatu." 86522. The World Bank.

Asian Development Bank. 2014. "The State of Pacific Towns and Cities. Urbanization in ADB's Pacific Developing Member Countries." www10.iadb.org/intal/intalcdi/PE/2012/07773 .pdf. Accessed December 10 2014.

Austin, J. L. 1962. *How to Do Things with Words*. Oxford, United Kingdom: Clarendon Press.

Bacon, Hannah. 2015. "Fat, Syn, and Disordered Eating: The Dangers and Powers of Excess." *Fat Studies* 4(2): 92–111.

Baer, Hans, Merrill Singer, and John Johnsen. 1986. "Introduction: Toward a Critical Medical Anthropology." *Social Science & Medicine* 23(2): 95–98.

Baer, Hans A., Merrill Singer, and Ida Susser. 2003. "Medical Anthropology: Central Concepts and Development." In *Medical Anthropology and the World System*. Second Edition. Pp. 3–30. Westport, CT: Praeger.

Baglar, Rosslyn. 2013. "'Oh God, Save Us from Sugar': An Ethnographic Exploration of Diabetes Mellitus in the United Arab Emirates." *Medical Anthropology* 32(2): 109–125.

Baker, Paul T., Joel M. Hanna, and Thelma S. Baker. 1986. *The Changing Samoans: Behavior and Health in Transition*. New York, NY: Oxford University Press.

Balkau, B., H. King, P. Zimmet, and L. R. Raper. 1985. "Factors Associated with the Development of Diabetes in the Micronesian Population of Nauru." *American Journal of Epidemiology* 122(4): 594–605.

Barker, Holly, and Rochelle Tuitagava'a Fonoti. 2010. "Collaboration and Capacity Building in the Classroom: A Decolonizing Teaching Agenda to Create a Cadre of Indigenous Researchers." *Pacific Studies* 33(2/3): 301–319.

Barnes, Shawn S., Darragh C. O'Carroll, Lauren Sumida, Leigh Anne Shafer, and Seiji Yamada. 2010. "Evidence for a Continuing Gap in Rural/Urban Adult Obesity in the Samoan Archipelago." *Journal of Community Health* 36(4): 534–537.

Bashkow, Ira. 2006. *The Meaning of Whiteman: Race and Modernity in the Orokaiva Cultural World*. Chicago, IL: University of Chicago Press.

Bauman, Richard. 1984. *Let Your Words Be Few: Symbolism and Silence among Seventeenth-Century Quakers*. Cambridge: Cambridge University Press.

Becker, Anne E. 1995. *Body, Self and Society: The View from Fiji*. Philadelphia, PA: University of Pennsylvania Press.

Becker, Anne E. 2004. "Television, Disordered Eating and Young Women in Fiji: Negotiating Body Image and Identity During Rapid Social Change." *Culture, Medicine and Psychiatry* 28(4): 533–559.

Becker, Gay. 1994. "Metaphors in Disrupted Lives: Infertility and Cultural Constructions of Continuity." *Medical Anthropology Quarterly* 8(4): 383–410.

Becker, Gay. 1997. *Disrupted Lives: How People Create Meaning in a Chaotic World*. Berkeley, CA: University of California Press.

Becker, Gay, Yewoubdar Beyene, Edwina Newsom, and Denise Rodgers. 1998. "Knowledge and Care of Chronic Illness in Three Ethnic Minority Groups." *Family Medicine* 30(3): 173–178.

Becker, Gay, Jan Rahima Gates, and Edwina Newsome. 2004. "Self-Care Among Chronically Ill African Americans: Culture, Health Disparities, and Health Insurance Status." *American Journal of Public Health* 94(12): 2066–2073.

Bell, Kristen, Darlene McNaughton, and Amy Salmon. 2011. *Alcohol, Tobacco and Obesity: Morality, Mortality and the New Public Health*. New York, NY: Routledge.

Berkman, L. F., T. Glass, I. Brissette, and T. E. Seeman. 2000. "From Social Integration to Health: Durkheim in the New Millennium." *Social Science & Medicine* 51(6): 843–857.

Berlant, Lauren. 2007. "Slow Death (Sovereignty, Obesity, Lateral Agency)." *Critical Inquiry* 33(4): 754–780.

Besnier, Niko. 2011. "Reconfiguring the Modern Christian." In *On the Edge of the Global: Modern Anxieties in a Pacific Island Nation*. Pp. 205–230. Stanford, CA: Stanford University Press.

Besnier, Niko. 2012. "The Athlete's Body and the Global Condition: Tongan Rugby Players in Japan." *American Ethnologist* 39(3): 491–510.

Bialecki, Jon. 2009. "Disjuncture, Continental Philosophy's New 'Political Paul,' and the Question of Progressive Christianity in a Southern California Third Wave Church." *American Ethnologist* 36(1): 110–123.

Bialecki, Jon. 2017. *A Diagram for Fire: Miracles and Variation in an American Charismatic Movement*. Berkeley, CA: University of California Press.

Biehl, João, and Adriana Petryna. 2013. *When People Come First: Critical Studies in Global Health*. Princeton, NJ: Princeton University Press.

Bielo, James. 2011. *Emerging Evangelicals*. New York, NY: New York University Press.

Bielo, James. 2014. "Act Like Men: Social Engagement and Evangelical Masculinity." *Journal of Contemporary Religion* 29(2): 233–248.

Biltekoff, Charlotte. 2013. *Eating Right in America: The Cultural Politics of Food and Health*. Durham, NC: Duke University Press.

Bindon, James, Douglas E. Crews, and William W. Dressler. 1991. "Life Style, Modernization and Adaptation Among Samoans." *Collegium Antropolgicum* 15(1): 101–110.

Bindon, James, Amy Knight, William W. Dressler, and Douglas E. Crews. 1997. "Social Context and Psychosocial Influences on Blood Pressure among American Samoans." *American Journal of Physical Anthropology* 10(3): 7–18.

Bloomer, Richard J., Trint A. Gunnels, and John Henry M. Schriefer. 2015. "Comparison of a Restricted and Unrestricted Vegan Diet Plan with a Restricted Omnivorous Diet Plan on Health-Specific Measures." *Healthcare* 3(3): 544–555.

Bloomer, Richard J., Mohammad M. Kabir, John F. Trepanowski, Robert E. Canale, and Tyler M. Farney. 2011. "A 21 Day Daniel Fast Improves Selected Biomarkers of Antioxidant Status and Oxidative Stress in Men and Women." *Nutrition and Metabolism* 8(17): 1–9.

Bloomer, Richard J., John F. Trepanowski, Mohammad M. Kabir, Rick J. Alleman, and Michael E. Dessoulavy. 2012. "Impact of Short-Term Dietary Modification on Postprandial Oxidative Stress." *Nutrition Journal* 11(16): 1–9.

Boero, Natalie. 2013. *Killer Fat: Media, Medicine, and Morals in the American "Obesity Epidemic."* New Brunswick, NJ: Rutgers University Press.

Bohannan, Paul. 1955. "Some Principles of Exchange and Investment Among the Tiv." *American Anthropologist* 57(1): 60–70.

Bordo, Susan. 1993. *Unbearable Weight: Feminism, Western Culture, and the Body*. Berkeley, CA: University of California.

Borovoy, Amy, and Janet Hine. 2008. "Managing the Unmanageable: Elderly Russian Jewish Emigres and the Biomedical Culture of Diabetes Care." *Medical Anthropology Quarterly* 22(1): 1–26.

Boyd, Mary. 1980. "Coping with Samoan Resistance after 1918 Influenza Epidemic." *Journal of Pacific History* 15(3): 155–174.

Brewis, Alexandra. 2011. *Obesity: Cultural and Biocultural Perspectives*. New Brunswick, NJ: Rutgers University Press.

Brewis, Alexandra, and Stephan McGarvey. 2000. "Body Image, Body Size and Samoan Ecological and Individual Modernization." *Ecology of Food and Nutrition* 39(2): 105–120.

Brewis, Alexandra, Stephen McGarvey, and B. A. Swinburn. 1998. "Perceptions of Body Size in Pacific Islanders." *International Journal of Obesity* 22: 185–189.

Brewis, Alexandra, Sarah Trainer, SeungYong Han, and Amber Wutich. 2016. "Publically Misfitting: Extreme Weight and the Everyday Production and Reinforcement of Felt Stigma." *Medical Anthropology Quarterly* 31(2): 257–276.

Brewis, Alexandra, Amber Wutich, Ashlan Falletta-Cowden, and Isa Rodriguez-Soto. 2011. "Body Norms and Fat Stigma in Global Perspective." *Current Anthropology* 52(2): 269–276.

Broom, Dorothy and Andrea Whittaker. 2004. "Controlling Diabetes, Controlling Diabetics: Moral Language in the Management of Diabetes Type 2." *Social Science & Medicine* 58(11): 2371–2382.

Brown, Richard P. C., and Dennis A. Ahlburg. 1999. "Remittances in the South Pacific." *International Journal of Social Economics* 26(1/2/3): 325–344.

Brownell, K. D., and D. Yach. 2006. "Lessons from a Small Country about the Global Obesity Crisis." *Globalization and Health* 2(11): 1–2.

Brusco, E. E. 1995. *The Reformation of Machismo: Evangelical Conversion and Gender in Columbia*. Austin, TX: University of Texas Press.

Burchardt, Marian. 2015. *Faith in the Time of AIDS - Religion, Biopolitics*. Basingstoke, United Kingdom: Palgrave.

Butler, Judith. 1993. *Bodies That Matter: On the Discursive Limits of "Sex."* New York, NY: Routledge.

Canaway, Rachel, and Lenore Manderson. 2013. "Quality of Life, Perceptions of Health and Illness, and Complementary Therapy Use among People with Type 2 Diabetes and Cardiovascular Disease." *Journal of Alternative and Complementary Medicine* 19(11): 882–890.

Capstick, Stuart, Pauline Norris, Faafetai Sopoaga, and Wale Tobata. 2009. "Relationships between Health and Culture in Polynesia—A Review." *Social Science & Medicine* 68(7): 1341–1348.

Carney, Megan. 2015a. *The Unending Hunger: Tracing Women and Food Insecurity Across Borders*. Berkeley, CA: University California Press.

Carney, Megan. 2015b. "Eating and Feeding at the Margins of the State: Barriers to Health Care for Undocumented Migrant Women and the 'Clinical' Aspects of Food Assistance." *Medical Anthropology Quarterly* 29(2): 196–215.

Carr, E. Summerson. 2015. "Occupation Bedbug: Or, the Urgency and Agency of Professional Pragmatism." *Cultural Anthropology* 30(2): 257–285.

Cassaniti, Julia. 2012. "Agency and the Other: The Role of Agency for the Importance of Belief in Buddhist and Christian Traditions." *Ethos* 40(3): 297–316.

Cassel, Kevin D. 2010. "Using the Social-Ecological Model as a Research and Intervention Framework to Understand and Mitigate Obesogenic Factors in Samoan Populations." *Ethnicity and Health* 15(4): 397–416.

Cassels, Susan. 2006. "Overweight in the Pacific: Links between Foreign Dependence, Global Food Trade, and Obesity in the Federated States of Micronesia." *Globalization and Health* 2 (July): 10.

Caton, Hiram. 1990. *The Samoa Reader: Anthropologists Take Stock*. Lanham, MD: University Press of America.

Centers for Disease Control and Prevention. 2017. "National Diabetes Statistics Report 2017: Estimates of Diabetes and Its Burden in the United States." Helmstedt, Germany: Centers for Disease Control and Prevention.

Choy, Courtney C., Mayur M. Desai, Jennifer J. Park, Elizabeth A. Frame, Avery A. Thompson, Take Naseri, Muagututia S. Reupena, Rachel L. Duckham, Nicole C. Deziel, and Nicola L. Hawley. 2017. "Child, Maternal and Household-Level Correlates of Nutritional Status: A Cross-Sectional Study among Young Samoan Children." *Public Health Nutrition* 20(7): 1235–1247.

Clark, Geoffrey. 2003. "Dumont d'Urville's Oceania." *The Journal of Pacific History* 38(2): 155–161.

Clarke, Laura Hurd, and Erica Bennett. 2013. "Constructing the Moral Body: Self-Care among Older Adults with Multiple Chronic Conditions." *Health* 17(3): 211–228.

Cobb, Sidney. 1976. "Social Support as a Moderator of Life Stress." *Psychosomatic Medicine* 38(5): 300–314.

Cole, Jennifer. 2012. "The Love of Jesus Never Disappoints: Reconstituting Female Personhood in Urban Madagascar." *Journal of Religion in Africa* 42(4): 384–407.

Coleman, Simon. 2000. *The Globalisation of Charismatic Christianity: Spreading the Gospel of Prosperity*. Cambridge, United Kingdom: Cambridge University Press.

Cooper, C. 2007. Headless Fatties. http://charlottecooper.net/fat/fat-writing/headless-fatties -01-07/

Corwin, Anna. 2012. "Changing God, Changing Bodies: The Impact of New Prayer Practices on Elderly Catholic Nuns' Embodied Experience." *Ethos* 40(4): 390–410.

Corwin, Anna. 2014. "Lord, Hear Our Prayer: Prayer, Social Support, and Well-Being in a Catholic Convent." *Journal of Linguistic Anthropology* 24(2): 174–192.

Corwin, Anna, and Jessica Hardin. Forthcoming. "Religion and Medicine: Productive Contrasts and Their Limitations." In *Oxford Handbook of the Anthropology of Religion*. Simon Coleman and Joel Robbins, eds.

Crawford, Robert. 1980. "Healthism and the Medicalization of Everyday Life." *International Journal of Health Services* 10(3): 365–388.

Crawford, Robert. 2006. "Health as a Meaningful Social Practice." *Health: An Interdisciplinary Journal for the Social Study of Health, Illness, and Medicine* 10(4): 401–420.

Csordas, Thomas J. 1983. "The Rhetoric of Transformation in Ritual Healing." *Culture, Medicine and Psychiatry* 7(4): 333–375.

Csordas, Thomas J. 1988. "Elements of Charismatic Persuasion and Healing." *Medical Anthropology Quarterly* 2(2): 445–469.

Csordas, Thomas J. 1993. "Somatic Modes of Attention." *Cultural Anthropology* 8(2): 135–156.

Csordas, Thomas J. 1994. *The Sacred Self: A Cultural Phenomenology of Charismatic Healing*. Berkeley, CA: University of California Press.

Csordas, Thomas J. 2002. *Body/Meaning/Healing*. New York, NY: Palgrave Macmillan.

de Montaigne, Michel. 2005. *On Friendship*. London, United Kingdom: Penguin UK.

Dein, Simon. 2002. "The Power of Words: Healing Narratives among Lubavitcher Hasidim." *Medical Anthropology Quarterly* 16(1): 41–63.

Diaz, Vicente, and J. Kehaulani Kauanui. 2001. "Native Pacific Culture Studies on the Edge." *The Contemporary Pacific* 13(2): 215–341.

Diez Roux, Ana V., and Christina Mair. 2010. "Neighborhoods and Health." *Annals of the New York Academy of Sciences* 1186: 125–145.

Dijk, Rijk van, Hansjörg Dilger, Marian Burchardt, and Thera Rasing, eds. 2014. *Religion and AIDS Treatment in Africa: Saving Souls, Prolonging Lives*. Surrey, United Kingdom: Ashgate Publishing, Ltd.

Doaks, C. M., L. Adair, M. Bentley, C. Monteiro, and B. M. Popkin. 2002. "The Nutrition Transition and Underweight/Overweight Household: A Seven Country Comparison." *FASEB Journal* 16(4): A615–A616.

Doucet-Battle, James. 2012. "Translating Sweetness: Type 2 Diabetes, Race, Research, and Outreach." Ph.D. Thesis. University of California, San Francisco.

Doucet-Battle, James. 2016. "Sweet Salvation: One Black Church, Diabetes Outreach, and Trust." *Transforming Anthropology* 24(2): 125–135.

Douglas, Mary. 1975. *Implicit Meanings: Selected Essays in Anthropology*. London, United Kingdom: Routledge.

Dressler, William W. 1980. "Coping Dispositions, Social Supports, and Health Status." *Ethos* 8(2): 146–171.

Dressler, William W., and James R. Bindon. 2000. "The Health Consequences of Cultural Consonance: Cultural Dimensions of Lifestyle, Social Support, and Arterial Blood Pressure in an African American Community." *American Anthropologist* 102(2): 244–260.

Du, Shufa, Thomas Mroz, Fengying Zhai, and Barry M. Popkin. 2004. "Rapid Income Growth Adversely Affects Diet Quality in China—Particularly for the Poor." *Social Science & Medicine* 59(7): 1505–1515.

Duranti, Alessandro. 1992. "Intentions, Self, and Responsibility: An Essay in Samoan Ethnopragmatics." In *Responsibility and Evidence in Oral Discourse*. Jane Hill and Judith T. Irvine, eds. Pp. 24–47. Cambridge, United Kingdom: Cambridge University Press.

Duranti, Alessandro. 1994. *From Grammar to Politics: Linguistic Anthropology in a Western Samoa Village*. Berkeley: University of California Press.

Dussart, Francoise. 2009. "Diet, Diabetes and Relatedness in a Central Australian Aboriginal Settlement: Some Qualitative Recommendations to Facilitate the Creation of Culturally Sensitive Health Promotion Initiatives." *Health Promotion Journal of Australia* 20(3): 202–206.

Dussart, Francoise. 2010. "'It Is Hard to Be Sick Now': Diabetes and the Reconstruction of Indigenous Sociality." *Anthropologica* 52(1): 77–87.

Eason, R. J., J. Pada, R. Wallace, A. Henry, and R. Thornton. 1987. "Changing Patterns of Hypertension, Diabetes, Obesity and Diet among Melanesians and Micronesians in the Solomon Islands." *The Medical Journal of Australia* 146(9): 465–469, 473.

Elisha, Omri. 2011. *Moral Ambitions: Mobilization and Social Outreach in Evangelical Megachurches*. Berkeley: University of California Press.

Ellison, Christopher G., and Jeffrey S. Levin. 1998. "The Religion-Health Connection: Evidence, Theory, and Future Directions." *Health Education & Behavior* 25(6): 700–720.

Elstad, Emily, Tusiofo Corabelle, Rochelle K. Rosen, and Stephen McGarvey. 2008. "Living with Ma'i Suka: Individual, Familial, Cultural, and Environmental Stress among Patients with Type 2 Diabetes Mellitus and Their Caregivers in American Samoa." *Preventing Chronic Disease* 5(3): 1–10.

Engelke, Matthew. 2004. "Discontinuity and the Discourse of Conversion." *Journal of Religion in Africa* 34(1): 82–109.

Engelke, Matthew. 2007. *A Problem of Presence: Beyond Scripture in an African Church*. Berkeley: University of California Press.

Engelke, Matthew. 2013. *God's Agents: Biblical Publicity in Contemporary England*. Berkeley: University of California Press.

Eriksen, Annelin. 2012. "The Pastor and the Prophetess: An Analysis of Gender and Christianity in Vanuatu." *Journal of the Royal Anthropological Institute* 18(1): 103–122.

Eriksen, Annelin. 2014. "Sarah's Sinfulness: Egalitarianism, Denied Difference, and Gender in Pentecostal Christianity." *Current Anthropology* 55(S10): S262–S270.

Ernst, Manfred. 2012. "Changing Christianity in Oceania: A Regional Overview." *Archives de Sciences Sociales Des Religions* 157(1): 29–45.

Errington, Frederick, and Deborah Gewertz. 2008. "Pacific Island Gastrologies: Following the Flaps." *Journal of the Royal Anthropological Institute* 14(3): 590–608.

Evans, M., R. C. Sinclair, C. Fusimalohi, and V. Liava'a. 2001. "Globalization, Diet, and Health: An Example from Tonga." *Bulletin of the World Health Organization* 79(9): 856–862.

Evans-Pritchard, E. E. 1937. *Witchcraft, Oracles, and Magic among the Azande*. Oxford, United Kingdom: Clarendon Press.

Eves, Richard. 2010. "'In God's Hands': Pentecostal Christianity, Morality, and Illness in a Melanesian Society." *Journal of the Royal Anthropological Institute* 16(3): 496–514.

Everett, Margaret, and Michelle Ramirez. 2015. "Healing the Curse of the Grosero Husband: Women's Health Seeking and Pentecostal Conversion in Oaxaca, Mexico." *Journal of Contemporary Religion* 30(3): 415–433.

Farmer, Paul. 2003. *Pathologies of Power: Health, Human Rights, and the New War on the Poor*. Berkeley: University of California Press.

Farmer, Paul, Jim Young Kim, Arthur Kleinman, and Matthew Basilico. 2013 *Reimaging Global Health: An Introduction*. Berkeley: University of California Press.

Fairbairn-Dunlop, Peggy. 1998. *Tamaitai Samoa: Their Stories*. Carson, CA: Institute of Pacific Studies.

Fee, Margaret. 2006. "Racializing Narratives: Obesity, Diabetes, and the 'Aboriginal Thrifty Genotype.'" *Social Science & Medicine* 62(12): 2988–2997.

Feld, Steven. 1982. *Sound and Sentiment: Birds, Weeping, Poetics, and Song in Kaluli Expression.* 2nd ed. Philadelphia: University of Pennsylvania Press.

Ferreira, Mariana Kawall Leal, and Gretchen Chesley Lang. 2006. *Indigenous Peoples and Diabetes: Community Empowerment and Wellness.* Durham, NC: Carolina Academic Press.

Ferry, Elizabeth. 2013. *Minerals, Collecting, and Value across the US-Mexico Border.* Bloomington, IN: University of Indiana Press.

Ferzacca, Steve. 2000. "'Actually, I Don't Feel That Bad': Managing Diabetes and the Clinical Encounter." *Medical Anthropology Quarterly* 14(1): 28–50.

Ferzacca, Steve. 2012. "Diabetes and Culture." *Annual Review of Anthropology* 41(1): 1–26.

Fessenden, Tracy. 2006. *Culture and Redemption: Religion, the Secular, and American Literature.* Princeton, NJ: Princeton University Press.

Fidler, D. 2004. *SARS, Governance and the Globalization of Disease.* Hampshire, UK: Springer.

Finkler, Kaja. 1984. *Spiritualist Healers in Mexico.* New York, NY: Praeger Publishers Inc.

Finkler, Kaja. 1994. "Sacred Healing and Biomedicine Compared." *Medical Anthropology Quarterly* 8(2): 178–197.

Finucane M. M., G. A. Stevens, M. J. Cowan, G. Danaei, J. K. Lin, C. J. Paciorek, G. M. Singh, H. R. Gutierrez, Y. Lu, A. N. Bahalim, F. Farzadfar, L. M. Riley, and M. Ezzati. 2011. "National, Regional, and Global Trends in Body-Mass Index Since 1980: Systematic Analysis of Health Examination Surveys and Epidemiological Studies with 960 Country-Years and 9.1 Million Participants." *Lancet* 377 (9765): 557–567.

Fischer, Edward F. 2014. *The Good Life: Aspiration, Dignity, and the Anthropology of Wellbeing.* Stanford, CA: Stanford University Press.

Fitzgerald, Thomas K. 1986. "Diet of Cook Islanders in New Zealand." In *Shared Wealth and Symbol: Food, Culture and Society in Oceania and Southeast Asia.* Lenore Manderson, ed. Pp. 67–86. Cambridge, United Kingdom: Cambridge University Press.

Freeman, Derek. 1983. *Margaret Mead and Samoa: The Making and Unmaking of an Anthropological Myth.* Cambridge, MA: Harvard University Press.

Freeman, Derek. 1991. "There's Tricks i' the' World: A Historical Analysis of the Samoan Researches of Margaret Mead." *Visual Anthropology Review* 7(1): 103–128.

Freeman, Derek. 1999. *The Fateful Hoaxing of Margaret Mead: A Historical Analysis of Her Samoan Research.* Boulder, CO: Westview Press.

Galanis, Daniel J., Stephen McGarvey, Christine Quested, Brenda Sio, and Salei 'a Afele-Fa'amuli. 1999. "Dietary Intake of Modernizing Samoans: Implications for Risk of Cardiovascular Disease." *Journal of American Dietetic Association* 99(2): 184–190.

Garro, Linda. 1995. "Individual or Societal Responsibility? Explanations of Diabetes in an Anishinaabe (Ojibway) Community." *Social Science & Medicine* 40(1): 37–46.

Garro, Linda. 2010. "Beyond the Reproduction of Official Accounts: Parental Commentary about Health and the Daily Life of a California Family." *Medical Anthropology Quarterly* 24(4): 472–499.

Garro, Linda, and Chesley Lang. 1993. "Explanations of Diabetes: Anishinaabeg and Dakota Deliberate upon a New Illness." In *Diabetes as a Disease of Civilization: The Impact of Culture Change on Indigenous Peoples.* Jennie R. Joe and Robert S. Young, eds. Pp. 293–328. Berlin, Germany: De Gruyter Mouton.

Gerber, Eleanor Ruth. 1985. "Rage and Obligation: Samoan Emotion in Conflict." In *Person, Self and Experience: Exploring Pacific Ethnopsychologies.* Geoffrey M. White and John Kirkpatrick, eds. Pp. 121–167. Berkeley: University of California Press.

Gerber, Lynne. 2012. *Seeking the Straight and Narrow: Weight Loss and Sexual Reorientation in Evangelical America*. Chicago, IL: University of Chicago Press.

Gerber, Lynne. 2015. "The Christian Dieter's Dilemma: Abundance and Restriction in Two Christian Weight Loss Programs." *Fat Studies* 4(2): 127–140.

Gerber, Lynne, Susan Hill, and LeRhonda Manigault-Bryant. 2015. "Religion and Fat = Protestant Christianity and Weight Loss? On the Intersections of Fat Studies and Religious Studies." *Fat Studies* 4(2): 82–91.

Gershon, Ilana. 2000. "How to Know When Not to Know: Strategic Ignorance When Eliciting for Samoan Migrant Exchanges." *Social Analysis* 44(2): 84–105.

Gershon, Ilana. 2006. "Converting Meanings and the Meanings of Conversion in Samoan Moral Economies." In *The Limits of Meaning: Case in the Anthropology of Christianity*. Matthew Engelke and Matt Tomlinson, eds. Pp. 147–164. New York, NY: Berghahn Books.

Gershon, Ilana. 2010. *The Breakup 2.0: Disconnecting over New Media*. Ithaca, NY: Cornell University Press.

Gershon, Ilana. 2011. "Neoliberal Agency." *Current Anthropology* 52(4): 537–555.

Gewertz, Deborah, and Frederick Errington. 2007. "The Alimentary Forms of the Global Life: The Pacific Island Trade in Lamb and Mutton Flaps." *American Anthropologist* 109(3): 496–508.

Gewertz, Deborah, and Frederick Errington. 2010. *Cheap Meat: Flap Food Nations in the Pacific Islands*. Berkeley: University of California Press.

Good, Byron J. 1994. *Medicine, Rationality, and Experience: An Anthropological Perspective*. New York, NY: Cambridge University Press.

Good, Mary. 2012. "'My Heart Is in the Phone': Romance and Mobile Morality." In *Modern Moralities, Moral Modernities: Ambivalence and Change Among Youth in Tonga*. Pp. 173–235. Ph.D. Thesis. Department of Anthropology, University of Arizona.

Golomski, Casey. 2014. "Generational Inversions: 'Working' for Social Reproduction amid HIV in Swaziland." *African Journal of AIDS Research* 13(4): 351–359.

Golomski, Casey. 2015a. "Compassion Technology: Life Insurance and the Remaking of Kinship in Swaziland's Age of HIV." *American Ethnologist* 42(1): 81–96.

Golomski, Casey. 2015b. "Wearing Memories: Clothing and the Global Lives of Mourning in Swaziland." *Material Religion* 11(3): 303–327.

Green, Linda. 2013. *Fear as a Way of Life: Mayan Widows in Rural Guatemala*. New York, NY: Columbia University Press.

Greenhalgh, Susan. 2012. "Weighty Subjects: The Biopolitics of the US War on Fat." *American Ethnologist* 39(3): 471–487.

Greenhalgh, Susan. 2015. *Fat-Talk Nation: The Human Costs of America's War on Fat*. Ithaca, NY: Cornell University Press.

Greenhalgh, Susan, and Megan Carney. 2014. "Bad Biocitizens?: Latinos and the US 'Obesity Epidemic.'" *Human Organization* 73(3): 267–276.

Gregory, C. A. 1997. *Savage Money: The Anthropology and Politics of Commodity Exchange*. Amsterdam, Netherlands: Harwood Academic.

Gremillion, Helen. 2005. "The Cultural Politics of Body Size." *Annual Review of Anthropology* 34: 13–32.

Griffith, R. Marie. 1997. *God's Daughters: Evangelical Women and the Power of Submission*. Berkeley: University of California Press.

Griffith, R. Marie. 2004. *Born Again Bodies: Flesh and Spirit in American Christianity*. Berkeley: University of California Press.

Guell, Cornelia. 2012. "Self-Care at the Margins: Meals and Meters in Migrants' Diabetes Tactics." *Medical Anthropology Quarterly* 26(4): 518–533.

Guthman, Julie. 2011. *Weighing In: Obesity, Food Justice, and the Limits of Capitalism.* Berkeley: University of California Press.

Guthman, Julie, and Melanie DuPuis. 2006. "Embodying Neoliberalism: Economy, Culture, and the Politics of Fat." *Environment and Planning: Society and Space* 24(3): 427–448.

Hamdy, Sherine. 2008. "When the State and Your Kidneys Fail: Political Etiologies in an Egyptian Dialysis Ward." *American Ethnologist* 35(4): 553–589.

Handman, Courtney. 2015. *Critical Christianity: Translation and Denominational Conflict in Papua New Guinea.* Berkeley: University of California Press.

Hardin, Jessica. 2013. "Fasting for Health, Fasting for God: Samoan Evangelical Christian Responses to Obesity and Chronic Disease." In *Reconstructing Obesity: The Measures of Meaning, the Meaning of Measures.* Megan McCullough and Jessica A. Hardin, eds. Pp. 107–130. New York, NY: Berghahn Books.

Hardin, Jessica. 2015a. "Everyday Translation: Health Practitioners' Perspectives on Obesity and Metabolic Disorders in Samoa." *Critical Public Health* 25(2): 125–138.

Hardin, Jessica. 2015b. "Christianity, Fat Talk, and Samoan Pastors: Rethinking the Fat-Positive-Fat-Stigma Framework." *Fat Studies* 4(2): 178–196.

Hardin, Jessica. 2016a. "'Healing Is a Done Deal': Temporality and Metabolic Healing among Evangelical Christians in Samoa." *Medical Anthropology* 35(2): 105–118.

Hardin, Jessica. 2016b. "Claiming Pule, Manifesting Mana: Ordinary Ethics and Pentecostal Self-Making in Samoa." In *New Mana: Re-Theorizing Mana across the Pacific.* Matt Tomlinson and Ty P. Kāwika Tengan, eds. Pp. 257–284. Canberra, Australia: ANU E Press.

Hardin, Jessica. 2016c. "Challenging Authority, Averting Risk, Creating Futures: Intersectionality and Interpreting Christian Ritual in Samoa." *Journal of Contemporary Religion* 31(3): 379–391.

Hardin, Jessica, and Christina Ting Kwauk. 2015. "Producing Markets, Producing People: Local Food, Financial Prosperity and Health in Samoa." *Food, Culture and Society* 18(3): 519–539.

Harding, Susan. 1987. "Convicted by the Holy Spirit: The Rhetoric of Fundamental Baptist Conversion." *American Ethnologist* 14(1): 167–181.

Harding, Susan. 1991. "Representing Fundamentalism: The Problem of the Repugnant Cultural Other." *Social Research* 58(2): 373–393.

Harding, Susan. 2000. *The Book of Jerry Falwell: Fundamentalist Language and Politics.* Princeton, NJ: Princeton University Press.

Harris, Stewart B., Jordan W. Tompkins, and Braden TeHiwi. 2016. "Call to Action: A New Path for Improving Diabetes Care for Indigenous Peoples, A Global Review." *Diabetes Research and Clinical Practice.* https://www.diabetesresearchclinicalpractice.com/article/S0168-8227(16)30246-7/abstract.

Harvey, Idethia Shevon, and Lawanda Cook. 2010. "Exploring the Role of Spirituality in Self-Management Practices among Older African-American and Non-Hispanic White Women with Chronic Conditions." *Chronic Illness* 6(2): 111–124.

Hasu, Päivi. 2006. "World Bank and Heavenly Bank in Poverty and Prosperity: The Case of Tanzanian Faith Gospel." *Review of African Political Economy* 33(110): 679–692.

Hau'ofa, Epeli. 1994. "Our Sea of Islands." *The Contemporary Pacific.* 6(1): 148–161.

Hawley, Nicola L., Ryan L. Minster, Daniel E. Weeks, Satupaitea Viali, Muagututia Sefuiva Reupena, Guangyun Sun, Hong Cheng, Ranjan Deka, and Stephen T. Mcgarvey. 2014. "Prevalence of Adiposity and Associated Cardiometabolic Risk Factors in the Samoan Genome-Wide Association Study." *American Journal of Human Biology* 26(4): 491–501.

Haynes, Naomi. 2012. "Pentecostalism and the Morality of Money: Prosperity, Inequality, and Religious Sociality on the Zambian Copperbelt." *Journal of the Royal Anthropological Institute* 18(1): 123–139.

Haynes, Naomi. 2013. "On the Potential and Problems of Pentecostal Exchange." *American Anthropologist* 115(1): 85–95.

Haynes, Naomi. 2017. *Moving by the Spirit: Pentecostal Social Life on the Zambian Copperbelt.* Berkeley: University of California Press.

Heard, Emma Marie, Leveti Auvaa, and Brooke A. Conway. 2016. "Culture X: Addressing Barriers to Physical Activity in Samoa." *Health Promotion International* 32(4): 734–742.

Held, Rachel Forster, Judith Rochelle DePue, Rochelle Rosen, Nicole Bereolos, Ofeira Nu'usolia, John Tuitele, Michael Goldstein, Meaghan House, and Stephen McGarvey. 2009. "Patient and Healthcare Provider Views of Depression and Diabetes in American Samoa." *Cultural Diversity and Ethnic Minority Psychology* 16(4): 461–467.

Henderson, April K. 2010. "Gifted Flows: Making Space for a Brand New Beat." *The Contemporary Pacific* 22(2): 293–315.

Hereniko, Vilsoni. 2000. "Indigenous Knowledge and Academic Imperialism." In *Remembrance of Pacific Pasts: An Invitation to Remake History.* Robert Borofsky, ed. Pp. 78–91. Honolulu: University of Hawaii Press.

Heron, Melonie. 2016. *National Vital Statistics Reports.* Hyattsville, MD: Centers for Disease Control and Prevention.

Hesse-Biber, S. 1997. *Am I Thin Enough Yet?: The Cult of Thinness and the Commercialization of Identity.* New York NY: Oxford University Press.

Hill, Samuel. 1985. *The South and the North in American Religion.* Athens: University of Georgia Press.

Hill, Susan E. 2011. *Eating to Excess: The Meaning of Gluttony and the Fat Body in the Ancient World.* Santa Barbara, CA: Praeger.

Hirschkind, Charles. 2006. *The Ethical Soundscape: Cassette Sermons and Islamic Counterpublics.* New York, NY: Columbia University Press.

Hodge, A. M., G. K. Dowse, P. Toelupe, V. R. Collins, and P. Z. Zimmet. 1994. "Dramatic Increase in the Prevalence of Obesity in Western Samoa over the 13 Year Period 1978–1991." *International Journal of Obesity* 18(6): 419–428.

Hojjat, Tahereh Alavi, and Rata Hojjat. 2017. *The Economics of Obesity: Poverty, Income Inequality and Health.* Berlin, Germany: Springer.

Hruschka, Daniel J. 2012. "Do Economic Constraints on Food Choice Make People Fat? A Critical Review of Two Hypotheses for the Poverty-Obesity Paradox." *American Journal of Human Biology: The Official Journal of the Human Biology Council* 24(3): 277–285.

Hunt, Linda M., Miguel A. Valenzuela, and Jacqueline A. Pugh. 1998. "Porque Me Tocó a Mi? Mexican American Diabetes Patients' Causal Stories and Their Relationship to Treatment Behaviors." *Social Science & Medicine* 46(8): 959–969.

Inhorn, Marcia. 2012. *The New Arab Man: Emergent Masculinities, Technologies, and Islam in the Middle East.* Princeton, NJ: Princeton University Press.

Inhorn, Marcia, and Soraya Tremayne. 2012. *Islam and Assisted Reproductive Technologies: Sunni and Shia Perspectives.* New York, NY: Berghahn.

Inhorn, Marcia, and Emily Wentzell. 2012. *Medical Anthropology at the Intersections: Histories, Activisms, and Futures.* Durham, NC: Duke University Press.

Izquierdo, Carolina. 2005. "When 'Health' Is Not Enough: Societal, Individual, and Biomedical Assessments of Well-Being among the Matsigenka of the Peruvian Amazon." *Social Science & Medicine* 61(4): 767–783.

Jacobs, Harrison. "The 10 Fattest Countries in the World. Business Insider." www.businessinsider.com/the-10-fattest-countries-in-the-world-2014-11. Accessed May 23, 2016.

Janes, Craig R. 1990. *Migration, Social Change, and Health: A Samoan Community in Urban California.* Stanford, CA: Stanford University Press.

Jehn, Megan, and Alexandra Brewis. 2009. "Paradoxical Malnutrition in Mother-Child Pairs: Untangling the Phenomenon of Over- and Under-Nutrition in Underdeveloped Economies." *Economics and Human Biology* 7(1): 28–35.

Jezewski, Mary Ann, and Jane Poss. 2002. "Mexican Americans' Explanatory Model of Type 2 Diabetes." *Western Journal of Nursing Research* 24(8): 840–858.

Jolly, Margaret. 2007. "Imagining Oceania: Indigenous and Foreign Representations of Sea of Islands." *The Contemporary Pacific* 19(2): 208–545.

Jutel, Annemarie. 2006. "The Emergence of Overweight as a Disease Entity: Measuring up Normality." *Social Science & Medicine* 63(9): 2268–2276.

Jutel, Annemarie. 2009. "Doctor's Orders: Diagnosis, Medical Authority and the Exploitation of the Fat Body." In *Biopolitics and the "Obesity Epidemic": Governing Bodies*. Jan Wright and Valerie Harwood, eds. Pp. 60–77. New York, NY: Routledge.

Kahn, Miriam. 1986. *Always Hungry, Never Greedy: Food and the Expression of Gender in a Melanesian Society*. Long Grove, IL: Waveland Press, Inc.

Kahn, Miriam, and Lorraine Sexton, eds. 1988. "Continuity and Change in Pacific." *Foodways* 3(1–2): 1–174.

Ka'ili, Tevita O. 2005. "Tauhi va: Nuturing Tongan Sociospatial Ties in Maui and Beyond." *The Contemporary Pacific* 17(1): 83–114.

Kameʻeleihiwa, Lilikalā. 1992. *Native Land and Foreign Desires: Pehea Lā E Pono Ai? How Shall We Live in Harmony?* Honolulu, HI: Bishop Museum Press.

Keane, Webb. 1997a. "From Fetishism to Sincerity: On Agency, the Speaking Subject, and Their Historicity in the Context of Religious Conversion." *Comparative Studies in Society and History* 39(4): 674–693.

Keane, Webb. 1997b. "Religious Language." *Annual Review of Anthropology* 26: 47–71.

Keane, Webb. 2007. *Christian Moderns: Freedom and Fetish in the Mission Encounter*. Berkeley: University of California Press.

Keck, Lois. 1994. "Social Networks and Support Groups: Experiences and Strategies for Managing a Chronic Disability." *Anthropology of Work Review* 15(23): 12–14.

Keighley, Ember D., Stephen McGarvey, Christine Quested, Charles McCuddin, Satupaitea Viali, Utoʻofili A. Maga, Ryutaro Ohtsuka, and Stanley J. Ulijaszek. 2007. "Nutrition and Health in Modernizing Samoans: Temporal Trends and Adaptive Perspectives." In *Health Changes in the Asia-Pacific Region: Biocultural and Epidemiological Approaches*. Ryutaro Ohtsuka and Stanley J. Ulijaszek, eds. Pp. 147–191. Cambridge, United Kingdom: Cambridge University Press.

Keshavjee, Salmaan. 2014. *Blind Spot: How Neoliberalism Infiltrated Global Health*. Berkeley: University of California Press.

Klaits, Frederick. 2010. *Death in a Church of Life: Moral Passion During Botswana's Time of AIDS*. Berkeley: University of California Press.

Klaits, Frederick. 2011. "Asking as Giving: Apostolic Prayers and the Aesthetics of Well-Being in Botswana." *Journal of Religion in Africa* 41(2): 206–226.

Klassen, Pamela. 2001a. "Sacred Maternities and Postbiomedical Bodies: Religion and Nature in Contemporary Home Birth." *Signs* 26(3): 775–809.

Klassen, Pamela. 2001b. *Blessed Events: Religion and Home Birth in America*. Princeton, NJ: Princeton University Press.

Klassen, Pamela. 2011. *Spirits of Protestantism: Medicine, Healing, and Liberal Christianity*. Berkeley, CA: University of California Press.

Klassen, Pamela. 2014. "The Politics of Protestant Healing: Theoretical Tools for the Study of Spiritual Bodies and The Body Politic." *Spiritus: A Journal of Christian Spirituality* 14(1): 68–75.

Kleinman, Arthur. 1978. "Culture, Illness, and Care: Clinical Lessons from Anthropologic and Cross-Cultural Research." *Annals of Internal Medicine* 88(2): 251–258.

Kleinman, Arthur. 1988. *Illness Narratives: Suffering, Healing and the Human Condition.* New York, NY: Basic Books.

Kleinman, Arthur. 1995. *Writing at the Margin: Discourse Between Anthropology and Medicine.* Berkeley: University of California Press.

Kleinman, Arthur. 2010. "Four Social Theories for Global Health." *The Lancet* 375(9725): 1518–1519.

Kleinman, Arthur, Veena Das, and Margaret Lock. 1997. *Social Suffering.* Berkeley: University of California Press.

Klingle, Matthew. 2015. "Inescapable Paradoxes: Diabetes, Progress, and Ecologies of Inequality." *Environmental History* 20(4): 736–750.

Klinken, Adriaan. 2012. "Men in the Remaking: Conversion Narratives and Born-Again Masculinity in Zambia." *Journal of Religion in Africa* 42(3): 215–239.

Kwauk, Christina Ting. 2006. "Goal! The Dream Begins: Globalizing an Immigrant Muscular Christianity." *Soccer and Society* 8(1): 75–89.

Kwauk, Christina Ting. 2014a. "Navigating Development Futures: Sport and the Production of Healthy Bodies in Samoa." Ph.D. Thesis. University of Minnesota.

Kwauk, Christina Ting. 2014b. "'No Longer Just a Pastime': Sport for Development in Times of Change." *The Contemporary Pacific* 26(2): 303–323.

Laderman, Carol, and Marina Roseman, eds. 1995. *The Performance of Healing.* New York, NY: Routledge.

Laidlaw, James. 2013. *The Subject of Virtue: An Anthropology of Ethics and Freedom.* Cambridge, United Kingdom: Cambridge University Press.

Lancet, The. 2016. "Beat Diabetes: An Urgent Call for Global Action." *The Lancet* 387(10027): 1483.

Landecker, Hannah. 2011. "Food as Exposure: Nutritional Epigenetics and the New Metabolism." *Biosocieties* 6(2): 167–194.

Lang, Chesley. 1989. "'Making Sense' About Diabetes: Dakota Narratives of Illness." *Medical Anthropology* 11(3): 305–327.

LeBesco, Kathleen. 2011. "Neoliberalism, Public Health, and the Moral Perils of Fatness." *Critical Public Health* 21(2): 153–164.

Lee, Helen Morton. 2003. *Tongans Overseas: Between Two Shores.* Honolulu: University of Hawaii Press.

Lee, Helen Morton, and Tupai Francis. 2009. *Migration and Transnationalism.* Canberra, Australia: ANU EPress.

Lesa, Mata'afa Keni. 2012a. "Change Begins with You and Me." *Samoa Observer.* January 3.

Lesa, Mata'afa Keni. 2012b. "Global Economy and Our Fa'alavelave." *Samoa Observer.* January 23.

Lester, Rebecca J. 2005. *Jesus in Our Wombs: Embodying Modernity in a Mexican Convent.* Berkeley: University of California Press.

Levi-Strauss, Claude. 1962. *The Savage Mind.* Chicago, IL: University of Chicago Press.

Li, Fuzhong, Peter Harmer, Bradley J. Cardinal, Mark Bosworth, and Deb Johnson-Shelton. 2009. "Obesity and the Built Environment: Does the Density of Neighborhood Fast-Food Outlets Matter?" *American Journal of Health Promotion* 23(3): 203–209.

Lieberman, Leslie Sue. 2003. "Dietary, Evolutionary, and Modernizing Influences on the Prevalence of Type 2 Diabetes." *Annual Review of Nutrition* 23(1): 345–377.

Likou, Lila. 2015. "Focus on Primary Health Care: Minister." *Samoa Observer.* June 6.

Lilomaiava-Doktor, Sa 'ilemanu. 2009. "Beyond 'Migration': Samoan Population Movement (Malaga) and the Geography of Social Space (Va)." *The Contemporary Pacific* 21(1): 1–32.

Lindquist, Galina, and Simon Coleman. 2008. "Against Belief?" *Social Analysis* 52(1): 1–18.

Lock, Margaret, and Ving-Kim Nguyen. 2010. *Anthropology of Biomedicine*. Malden, MA: Wiley-Blackwell.

Loewe, Ron, and Joshua Freeman. 2000. "Interpreting Diabetes Mellitus: Differences between Patient and Provider Models of Disease and Their Implications for Clinical Practice." *Culture, Medicine and Psychiatry* 24(4): 379–401.

Luhrmann, Tanya. 2012. *When God Talks Back: Understanding the American Evangelical Relationship with God*. New York, NY: Knopf.

Luhrmann, Tanya. 2013. "Making God Real and Making God Good: Some Mechanisms through Which Prayer May Contribute to Healing." *Transcultural Psychiatry* 50(5): 707–725.

Luhrmann, Tanya Marie, and Rachel Morgain. 2012. "Prayer as Inner Sense Cultivation: An Attentional Learning Theory of Spiritual Experience." *Ethos* 40(4): 359–389.

Lupton, Deborah. 2013. *Fat*. New York, NY: Routledge.

Macpherson, Cluny. 1985. "Samoan Medicine." In *Healing Practices in the South Pacific*. Claire D. F. Parsons, ed. Pp. 1–15. Honolulu, HI: The Institute for Polynesian Studies.

Macpherson, Cluny, and La 'avasa Macpherson. 1990. *Samoan Medical Belief and Practice*. Honolulu: University of Hawaii Press.

Macpherson, Cluny, and La 'avasa Macpherson. 2009. *The Warm Winds of Change: Globalization in Contemporary Samoa*. Auckland, New Zealand: Auckland University Press.

Macpherson, Cluny, and La 'avasa Macpherson. 2011. "Churches and the Economy of Samoa." *The Contemporary Pacific* 23(2): 304–337.

Mageo, Jeannette Marie. 1989. "Aga, Amio, and Loto: Perspectives on the Structure of the Self in Samoa." *Oceania* 59(3): 181–199.

Mageo, Jeannette Marie. 1998. *Theorizing Self in Samoa: Emotions, Genders and Sexualities*. Ann Arbor: The University of Michigan Press.

Mahoney, Carolyn. 2015. *Health, Food, and Social Inequality: Critical Perspectives on the Supply and Marketing of Food*. New York, NY: Routledge.

Mahmood, Saba. 2005. *The Politics of Piety: Islamic Revival and the Feminist Subject*. Princeton, NJ: Princeton University Press.

Manderson, Lenore. 1986. *Shared Wealth and Symbol: Food, Culture, and Society in Oceania and Southeast Asia*. Cambridge, United Kingdom: Cambridge University Press.

Manderson, Lenore. 2016. "Anthropological Perspectives on the Health Transition." In *International Encyclopedia of Public Health*. Second Edition. Pp. 122–128. Oxford, United Kingdom: Academic Press.

Manderson, Lenore, and Renata Kokanovic. 2009. "'Worried All the Time:' Distress and the Circumstances of Everyday Life among Immigrant Australians with Type 2 Diabetes." *Chronic Illness* 5(1): 21–32.

Manderson, Lenore, and Carolyn Smith-Morris. 2010. *Chronic Conditions, Fluid States: Chronicity and the Anthropology of Illness*. New Brunswick, NJ: Rutgers University Press.

Manderson, Lenore, and Narelle Warren. 2016. "'Just One Thing after Another': Recursive Cascades and Chronic Conditions." *Medical Anthropology Quarterly* 30(4): 479–497.

Manuela, S., and C. G. Sibley. 2015. "The Pacific Identity and Wellbeing Scale-Revised (PIWBS-R)." *Cultural Diversity and Ethnic Minority Psychology* 21(1): 146–155.

Marshall, Ruth. 2009. *Political Spiritualities: The Pentecostal Revolution in Nigeria*. Chicago, IL: University of Chicago Press.

Marshall, Wende Elizabeth. 2012a. *Potent Mana: Lessons in Power and Healing*. Albany, NY: SUNY Press.

Marshall, Wende Elizabeth. 2012b. "Tasting Earth: Healing, Resistance Knowledge, and the Challenge to Dominion." *Anthropology and Humanism* 37(1): 84–99.

Martin, Emily. 1987. *The Woman in the Body: A Cultural Analysis of Reproduction*. Boston, MA: Beacon Press.

Martin, Emily. 1991. "The Egg and the Sperm: How Science Has Constructed a Romance Based on Stereotypical Male-Female Roles." *Signs* 16(3): 485–501.

Mathews, Gordon, and Carolina Izquierdo. 2009. *Pursuits of Happiness: Well-Being in Anthropological Perspective*. New York, NY: Berghahn Books.

Mattingly, Cheryl, and Linda Garro. 2000. *Narrative and the Cultural Construction of Illness and Healing*. Berkeley: University of California Press.

Maxwell, David. 1998. "'Delivered from the Spirit of Poverty?': Pentecostalism, Prosperity, and Modernity in Zimbabwe." *Journal of Religion in Africa* 28(3): 350–373.

McClure, Stephanie. 2017. "Symbolic Body Capital of an 'Other' Kind: African American Females as a Bracketed Subunit in Female Body Valuation." In *Fat Planet: Obesity, Culture, and Symbolic Body Capital*. Eileen P. Anderson-Fye and Alexandra Brewis, eds. Pp. 97–124. Albuquerque, NM: University of New Mexico Press.

McCullough, Megan. 2013. "Fat and Knocked-Up: An Embodied Analysis of Stigma, Visibility and Invisibility in the Biomedical Management of an Obese Pregnancy." In *Reconstructing Obesity Research: The Measures of Meaning, the Meaning of Measures*. Megan McCullough and Jessica Hardin, eds. Pp. 215–234. New York, NY: Berghahn Books.

McCullough, Megan, and Jessica Hardin, eds. 2013. *Reconstructing Obesity: The Meaning of Measures and the Measure of Meanings*. New York, NY: Berghahn Books.

McDade, Thomas W. 2001. "Lifestyle Incongruity, Social Integration, and Immune Function in Samoan Adolescents." *Social Science & Medicine* 53(10): 1351–1362.

McDade, Thomas W. 2002. "Status Incongruity in Samoan Youth: A Bicultural Analysis of Culture Change, Stress, and Immune Function." *Medical Anthropology Quarterly* 16(2): 123–150.

McGarvey, Stephen. 1995. "Thrifty Genotype Concepts and Health in Modernizing Samoa." *Asia Pacific Journal of Clinical Nutrition* 4(4): 351–353.

McGarvey, Stephen, and Paul T. Baker. 1979. "The Effects of Modernization and Migration on Samoan Blood Pressures." *Human Biology* 51(4): 461–479.

McGarvey, Stephen, James Bindon, Douglas E. Crews, and Diana E. Schendel. 1989.

McGarvey, Stephan., and A. Seiden. 2010. "Health, Well-Being, and Social Context of Samoan Migrant Populations." *NAPA Bulletin* 34(1): 213–228.

McGrath, Barbara Burns. 1999. "Swimming from Island to Island: Healing Practice in Tonga." *Medical Anthropology Quarterly* 13(4): 483–505.

McKeown, Thomas. 1976. *The Modern Rise of Population*. London, United Kingdom: Academic Press.

McLaren, Lindsay. 2007. "Socioeconomic Status and Obesity." *Epidemiological Reviews* 29(1): 29–48.

McLennan, A. K., and S. J. Ulijaszek. 2015a. "An Anthropological Insight into the Pacific Island Diabetes Crisis and Its Clinical Implications." *Diabetes Management* 5(3):143–145.

McLennan, A. K., and S. J. Ulijaszek. 2015b. "Obesity Emergence in the Pacific Islands: Why Understanding Colonial History and Social Change Is Important." *Public Health Nutrition* 18(8): 1499–1505.

McLennan, Amy K. 2015. "Bringing Everyday Life into the Study of 'Lifestyle Diseases.' Lessons from an Ethnographic Investigation of Obesity Emergence in Nauru." *Journal of the Anthropological Society of Oxford* 7(3): 286–301.

McMullin, Juliet. 2005. "The Call to Life: Revitalizing a Healthy Hawaiian Identity." *Social Science & Medicine* 61: 809–820.

McMullin, Juliet. 2010. *The Healthy Ancestor: Embodied Inequality and the Revitalization of Native Hawaiian Health*. Walnut Creek, CA: Left Coast Press.

McNaughton, Darlene. 2011. "From Womb to the Tomb: Obesity and Maternal Responsibility." *Critical Public Health* 21(2): 179–190.

Mead, Margaret. 1928a. "The Role of the Individual in Samoan Culture." *The Journal of the Royal Anthropological Institute of Great Britain and Ireland* 58: 481–495.

Mead, Margaret. 1928b. *Coming of Age in Samoa: A Psychological Study of Primitive Youth for Western Civilization*. New York, NY: Perennial Classics.

Meleisea, Leasiolagi Malama. 1987. *The Making of Modern Samoa: Traditional Authority and Colonial Administration in the History of Western Samoa*. Suva, Fiji: Institute of Pacific Studies, University of the South Pacific.

Meleisea, Leasiolagi Malama. 1997. *The Cambridge History of the Pacific Islanders*. Cambridge, United Kingdom: Cambridge University Press.

Mendenhall, Emily. 2012. *Syndemic Suffering: Social Distress, Depression, and Diabetes among Mexican Immigrant Women*. Walnut Creek, CA: Left Coast Press.

Mendenhall, Emily, Alicia Fernandez, Nancy Adler, and Elizabeth A. Jacobs. 2012a. "Susto, Coraje, and Abuse: Depression and Beliefs about Diabetes." *Culture, Medicine, and Psychiatry* 36(3): 480–492.

Mendenhall, Emily, Rebecca A. Seligman, Alicia Fernandez, and Elizabeth A. Jacobs. 2010. "Speaking through Diabetes: Rethinking the Significance of Lay Discourse on Diabetes." *Medical Anthropology Quarterly* 24(2): 220–239.

Mendenhall, Emily, Roopa Shivashankar, Nikhil Tandon, K. Ali Mohammed, K.M.V. Narayan, and Prabhakaran Dorairaj. 2012b. "Stress and Diabetes in Socioeconomic Context: A Qualitative Study of Urban Indians." *Social Science & Medicine* 75(12): 2522–2529.

Mercado-Martinez, Francisco J., and Igor Martin Ramos-Herrera. 2002. "Diabetes: The Layperson's Theories of Causality." *Qualitative Health Research* 12(6): 792–806.

Merry, Sally Engle. 2016. *The Seductions of Quantification: Measuring Human Rights, Gender Violence, and Sex Trafficking*. Chicago, IL: University of Chicago Press.

Metzl, Jonathan M., and Anna Kirkland. 2010. *Against Health: How Health Became the New Morality*. New York, NY: New York University Press.

Meyer, Birgit. 1998. "Commodities and the Power of Prayer. Pentecostalist Attitudes Towards Consumption in Contemporary Ghana." *Development and Change* 29(4): 751–776.

Meyer, Birgit. 2011. "Mediation and Immediacy: Sensational Forms, Semiotic Ideologies, and the Question of the Medium." *Social Anthropology* 19(1): 23–39.

Miller, Daniel. 2005. *Materiality*. Durham, NC: Duke University Press.

Minster, Ryan, Nicola L. Hawley, Chi-Ting Su, Guangyun Sun, Erin E. Kershaw, Hong Cheng, Olive D. Buhule, Jerome Lin, Muagututi'a Sefuiva Reupena, Satupa'itea Viali, John Tuitele, Take Naseri, Zsolt Urban, Ranjan Deka, Daniel E. Weeks, and Stephen T. McGarvey. 2016. "A Thrifty Variant in CREBRF Strongly Influences Body Mass Index in Samoans." *Nature Genetics* 48(9): 1049–1054.

Ministry of Health. 2010. *National Non-communicable Disease Policy 2010–2015*. Apia, Samoa: Government of Samoa.

Ministry of Health. 2012. *Corporate Plan 2013–2016*. Apia, Samoa.

Mitchem, Stephanie. 2007. *African American Folk Healing*. New York, NY: New York University Press.

Mitchem, Stephanie. 2010. *African American Women Tapping Power and Spiritual Wellness*. Eugene, OR: Wipf and Stock Publishers.

Miyazaki, Hirokazu. 2000. "Faith and Fulfillment: Agency, Exchange, and the Fijian Aesthetics of Completion." *American Ethnologist* 27(1): 31–51.

"Modernization and Adiposity: Causes and Consequences." In *Human Population Biology*. Michael Little and Haas D. Jere, eds. Pp. 263–280. Oxford, United Kingdom: Oxford University Press.

Mol, Annemarie. 2009. "Living with Diabetes: Care beyond Choice and Control." *The Lancet* 373(9677): 1756–1757.

Monteiro, Carlos A., Erly C. Moura, Wolney L. Conde, and Barry M. Popkin. 2004. "Socioeconomic Status and Obesity in Adult Populations of Developing Countries: A Review." *Bulletin of the World Health Organization* 82(12): 940–946.

Montesi, Laura. 2017. "'Como Si Nada': Enduring Violence and Diabetes among Rural Women in Southern Mexico." *Medical Anthropology* 37(3): 206–220.

Montoya, Michael. 2011. *Making the Mexican Diabetic: Race, Science, and the Genetics of Inequality*. Berkeley: University of California Press.

Moore, S. E., H. Y. Leslie, and C. A. Lavis. 2005. "Subjective Well-Being and Life Satisfaction in the Kingdom of Tonga." *Social Indicators Research* 70(3): 287–311.

Moyer, Eileen, and Anita Hardon. 2014. "A Disease Unlike Any Other? Why HIV Remains Exceptional in the Age of Treatment." *Medical Anthropology* 33(4): 263–269.

Moyle, Richard. 1974. "Samoan Medical Incantations." *Journal of Polynesian Society* 83(2): 155–179.

Munn, Nancy. 1986. *The Fame of Gawa: A Symbolic Study of Value Transformation in a Massim (Papua New Guinea) Society*. Durham, NC: Duke University Press.

Naemiratch, Bhensri, and Lenore Manderson. 2006. "Control and Adherence: Living with Diabetes in Bangkok, Thailand." *Social Science & Medicine* 63(5): 1147–1157.

Namageyo-Funa, Apophia, and Jessica Muilenburg. 2013. "The Role of Religion and Spirituality in Coping with Type 2 Diabetes: A Qualitative Study among Black Men." *Journal of Religion and Health* 54(1): 242–252.

Nanditha, Arun, Ronald C. W. Ma, Ambuddy Ramachandran, Chamukuttan Snehalatha, Juliana C. N. Chan, Kee Send Chia, Jonathan E. Shaw, and Paul Z. Zimmet. 2016. "Diabetes in Asia and the Pacific: Implications for the Global Epidemic." *Diabetes Care* 39(3): 472–485.

NCD Risk Factor Collaboration. 2016. "Trends in Adult Body-Mass Index in 200 Countries from 1975 to 2014: A Pooled Analysis of 1698 Population-Based Measurement Studies with 19.2 Million Participants." *The Lancet* 387(10026): 1377–1396.

Neel, James. 1962. "Diabetes Mellitus: A 'Thrifty' Genotypes Rendered Detrimental by 'Progress'?" *The American Journal of Human Genetics* 14(4): 353–362.

Nichter, Mimi. 2000. *Fat Talk: What Girls and Their Parents Say about Dieting*. Cambridge, MA: Harvard University Press.

Ochs, Elinor. 2004. "Narrative Lessons." In *A Companion to Linguistic Anthropology*. Alessandro Duranti, ed. Pp. 269–289. Malden, MA: Blackwell Publishing.

Olson, B. 2001. "Meeting the Challenges of American Indian Diabetes: Anthropological Perspectives on Treatment and Prevention." In *Medicine Ways: Disease, Health and Survival among Native Americans*. Clifford E. Trafzer and Diane E. Weiner, eds. Walnut Creek, CA: Alta Mira.

Omran, Abdel R. 1971. "The Epidemiologic Transition: A Theory of the Epidemiology of Population Change." *The Milbank Memorial Fund Quarterly* 49(4): 509–538.

Ortner, Sherry B. 2006. *Anthropology and Social Theory: Culture, Power, and the Acting Subject*. Durham, NC: Duke University Press.

Pagaialii, Tavita. 2006. *Pentecost "to the Uttermost": A History of the Assemblies of God in Samoa*. Baguio City, Philippines: APTS Press.

Panosian, Claire, and Thomas J. Coates. 2006. "The New Medical 'Missionaries'—Grooming the Next Generation of Global Health Workers." *New England Journal of Medicine* 354(17): 1771–1773.

Parmentier, Richard J. 2002. "Money Walks, People Talk: Systemic and Transactional Dimensions of Palauan Exchange." *L'Homme* 162(2): 49–80.

Parsons, Claire. 1985. *Healing Practices in the South Pacific*. Honolulu, HI: The Institute for Polynesian Studies.

Pellegrini, Ann, and Janet R. Jakobsen, eds. 2008. *Secularisms*. Durham, NC: Duke University Press Books.

Peña, Manuel, and Jorge Bacallao. 2000. *Obesity and Poverty: A New Public Health Challenge*. Washington, DC: Pan American Health Organization.

Pigg, Stacy Leigh. 2013. "On Sitting and Doing: Ethnography as Action in Global Health." *Social Science & Medicine* 99: 127–134.

Pitaloka, Dyah, and Elaine Hsieh. 2015. "Health as Submission and Social Responsibilities Embodied Experiences of Javanese Women with Type II Diabetes." *Qualitative Health Research* 25(8): 1155–1165.

Pollock, Nancy. 1985. "The Concept of Food in a Pacific Society: A Fijian Example." *Ecology of Food and Nutrition* 17(3): 195–203.

Pollock, Nancy. 1986. "Taro and Timber: Competing or Complementary Ways to a Food Supply." In *Shared Wealth and Symbol: Food, Culture and Society in Oceania and Southeast Asia*. Lenore Manderson, ed. Pp. 87–110. Cambridge, United Kingdom: Cambridge University Press.

Pollock, Nancy. 1992. *These Roots Remain: Food Habits in Islands of the Central and Eastern Pacific Since Western Contact*. Laie, HI: The Institute for Polynesian Studies.

Pollock, Nancy. 1995. "Cultural Elaborations of Obesity: Fattening Practices in Pacific Societies." *Asia Pacific Journal of Clinical Nutrition* 4: 357–360.

Pollock, Nancy. 2001. "Obesity or Large Body Size? A Study of Wallis and Futuna." *Pacific Health Dialog* 8(1): 119–123.

Pollock, Nancy. 2011. "The Language of Food." In *The Oxford Handbook of Linguistic Fieldwork*. Nicolas Thieberger and Nick Thieberger, eds. Pp. 235–249. Oxford: Oxford University Press.

Polzer, Rebecca L. 2007. "African Americans and Diabetes: Spiritual Role of the Health Care Provider in Self-Management." *Research in Nursing and Health* 30(2): 164–174.

Polzer, Rebecca L., and Margaret S. Miles. 2007. "Spirituality in African Americans with Diabetes: Self-Management through a Relationship with God." *Qualitative Health Research* 17(2): 176–188.

Popkin, Barry M. 1994. "The Nutrition Transition in Low-Income Countries: An Emerging Crisis." *Nutrition Reviews* 52(9): 285–298.

Popkin, Barry M. 2008. "Will China's Nutrition Transition Overwhelm Its Health Care System and Slow Economic Growth?" *Health Affairs* 27(4): 1064–1076.

Popkin, Barry M., Linda S. Adair, and Shu Wen Ng. 2012. "Global Nutrition Transition and the Pandemic of Obesity in Developing Countries." *Nutrition Reviews* 70(1): 3–21.

Popkin, Barry M., and P. Gordon-Larsen. 2004. "The Nutrition Transition: Worldwide Obesity Dynamics and Their Determinants." *International Journal of Obesity* 28: S2–S9.

Poss, Jane, and Mary Ann Jezewski. 2002. "The Role and Meaning of Susto in Mexican Americans' Explanatory Model of Type 2 Diabetes." *Medical Anthropology Quarterly* 16(3): 360–377.

Powdermaker, Hortense. 1960. "An Anthropological Approach to the Problem of Obesity." *Bulletin of the New York Academy of Medicine* 36(5): 286–295.

Prince, Ruth, Philippe Denis, and Rijk van Dijk. 2009. "Introduction to Special Issue: Engaging Christianities: Negotiating HIV/AIDS, Health, and Social Relations in East and Southern Africa." *Africa Today* 56(1): v–xviii.

Queensland Government. 2011. *Queensland Health Response to Pacific Islander and Māori Health Needs Assessment*. Brisbane, Australia: Division of the Chief Health Officer.

Rabinow, Paul. 2005. "Artificiality and Enlightenment: From Sociobiology to Biosociality." In *Anthropologies of Modernity*. Jonathan Xavier Inda, ed. Pp. 179–193. Malden, MA: Blackwell Publishing.

Richards, Fayana. 2014. "Field Notes: Care—Cultural Anthropology." Correspondences, Cultural Anthropology website. https://culanth.org/fieldsights/498-field-notes-care. Accessed May 11, 2017.

Robbins, Joel. 2001. "God Is Nothing but Talk: Modernity, Language, and Prayer in a Papua New Guinea Society." *American Anthropologist* 103(4): 901–912.

Robbins, Joel. 2004a. *Becoming Sinners: Christianity and Moral Torment in a Papua New Guinea Society*. Berkeley: University of California Press.

Robbins, Joel. 2004b. "The Globalization of Pentecostal and Charismatic Christianity." *Annual Review of Anthropology* 33: 117–143.

Robbins, Joel. 2007. "Continuity Thinking and the Problem of Christian Culture: Belief, Time, and the Anthropology of Christianity." *Current Anthropology* 48(1): 5–38.

Robbins, Joel. 2009. "Pentecostal Networks and the Spirit of Globalization: On the Social Productivity of Ritual Forms." *Social Analysis* 53(1): 55–66.

Robbins, Joel. 2012. "Spirit Women, Church Women, and Passenger Women." *Archives de Sciences Sociales des Religions* 157: 113–133.

Rock, Melanie. 2003. "Sweet Blood and Social Suffering: Rethinking Cause-Effect Relationships in Diabetes, Distress, and Duress." *Medical Anthropology* 22(2): 131–174.

Rose, Nikolas. 1999. *Powers of Freedom: Reframing Political Thought*. Cambridge, United Kingdom: Cambridge University Press.

Rose, Nikolas. 2000. "Government and Control." *British Journal of Criminology* 40 (2): 321–339.

Rosen, Rochelle K., Judith DePue, and Stephen McGarvey. 2008. "Overweight and Diabetes in American Samoa: The Cultural Translation of Research into Health Care Practice." *Medicine and Health/Rhode Island* 91(12): 372–377.

Rothblum, Esther, and Sondra Solovay, eds. 2009. *The Fat Studies Reader*. New York, NY: University Press.

Rubin, Lisa, and Jessica Joseph. 2013. "An Ounce of Prevention, a Ton of Controversy: Exploring Tensions in the Fields of Obesity and Eating Disorder Prevention." In *Reconstructing Obesity Research: The Measures of Meaning, the Meaning of Measures*. Megan McCullough and Jessica Hardin, eds. Pp. 199–214. New York, NY: Berghahn Books.

Saethre, Eirik. 2013. *Illness Is a Weapon: Indigenous Identity and Enduring Afflictions*. Nashville, TN: Vanderbilt University Press.

Saguy, Abigail. 2013. *What's Wrong with Fat?* New York, NY: Oxford University Press.

Saguy, Abigail C., and Rene Almeling. 2008. "Fat in the Fire? Science, the News Media, and the 'Obesity Epidemic.'" *Sociological Review* 23(1): 53–83.

Saguy, Abigail C., and Kevin W. Riley. 2005. "Weighing Both Sides: Morality, Mortality, and Framing Contests over Obesity." *Journal of Health Politics* 30(5): 869–921.

Salesa, Damon. 2011. *Racial Crossings: Race, Intermarriage and the Victorian British Empire*. Oxford, United Kingdom: Oxford University Press.

Samoa, Congregational Christian Church. N.d. Parishes. www.cccs.org.ws/index.php?option=com_content&view=category&layout=blog&id=37&Itemid=125.

Samoan Bureau of Statistics. 2012. *Population and Housing Census 2011*. Apia, Samoa.

Sanabria, Emilia. 2016. "Circulating Ignorance: Complexity and Agnogenesis in the Obesity 'Epidemic.'" *Cultural Anthropology* 31(1): 131–158.

Scheder, Jo. 1988. "A Sickly-Sweet Harvest: Farmworker Diabetes and Social Equality." *Medical Anthropology Quarterly* 2(3): 251–277.

Scheper-Hughes, Nancy, and Margaret Lock. 1987. "The Mindful Body: A Prolegomenon to Future Work in Medical Anthropology." *Medical Anthropology Quarterly* 1(1): 6–41.

Schoeffel, Penelope. 1984. "Dilemmas of Modernization in Primary Health Care in Western Samoa." *Social Science & Medicine* 19(3): 209–216.

Schoeffel, Penelope. 1994. "Social Change." In *Tides of History: The Pacific Islands in the Twentieth Century*. K. R. Howe, Robert C. Kiste, and Brij V. Lal, eds. St Leonard's, United Kingdom: Allen and Unwin.

Schoenberg, Nancy E., and Elaine M. Drew. 2002. "Articulating Silences: Experiential and Biomedical Constructions of Hypertension Symptomatology." *Medical Anthropology Quarterly* 16(4): 458–475.

Schoenberg, Nancy E., Elaine M. Drew, Eleanor Palo Stoller, and Cary S. Kart. 2005. "Situating Stress: Lessons from Lay Discourses on Diabetes." *Medical Anthropology Quarterly* 19(2): 171–193.

Schram, Ryan. 2013. "One Mind: Enacting the Christian Congregation among the Auhelawa, Papua New Guinea." *TAJA: The Australian Journal of Anthropology* 24(1): 30–47.

Schwarz, Carolyn. 2010. "Sick Again, Well Again: Sorcery, Christianity, and Kinship in Northern Aboriginal Australia." *Anthropological Forum* 20(1): 61–80.

Scrinis, Gyorgy. 2008. "On the Ideology of Nutritionism." *Gastronomica: The Journal of Critical Food Studies* 8(1): 39–48.

Seeberg, Jen, and Lotte Meinert. 2015. "Can Epidemics Be Noncommunicable? Reflections on the Spread of 'Noncommunicable' Diseases." *Medicine Anthropology Theory* 2(2): 54–71.

Seiden, Andrew, Nicola Hawley, Dirk Schulz, Sarah Raifman, and Stephen T. McGarvey. 2012. "Long-Term Trends in Food Availability, Food Prices, and Obesity in Samoa." *American Journal of Human Biology* 24(3): 286–295.

Seligman, Rebecca. 2010. "The Unmaking and Making of Self: Embodied Suffering and Mind–Body Healing in Brazilian Candomblé." *Ethos* 38(3): 297–320.

Seligman, Rebecca, Emily Mendenhall, Maria Valdovinos, Alicia Fernandez, and Elizabeth Jacobs. 2015. "Self-Care and Subjectivity among Mexican Diabetes Patients in the United States." *Medical Anthropology Quarterly* 29(1): 61–79.

Shankman, Paul. 2009. *The Trashing of Margaret Mead: Anatomy of an Anthropological Controversy*. Madison, WI: University of Wisconsin Press.

Shoaps, Robin A. 2002. "'Pray Earnestly': The Textual Construction of Personal Involvement in Pentecostal Prayer and Song." *Journal of Linguistic Anthropology* 12(1): 34–71.

Shore, Bradd. 1982. *Sala'ilua: A Samoan Mystery*. New York, NY: Columbia University Press.

Shore, Bradd. 1989. "Mana and Tapu." In *Developments in Polynesian Ethnology*. Alan Howard and Robert Borofsky, eds. Pp. 137–173. Honolulu: University of Hawaii Press.

Shore, Bradd. 1990. "Human Ambivalence and the Structuring of Moral Values." *Ethos* 18(2): 165–179.

Silva, Kalena. 1997. "The Adoption of Christian Prayer in Native Hawaiian Pule." *Pacific Studies* 20(1): 89–99.

Simmons, D. 1998. "A Pilot Urban Church-Based Programme to Reduce Risk Factors for Diabetes Among Western Samoans in New Zealand." *Diabetic Medicine* 15(2): 136–142.

Singer, Merrill. 2009. "Pathogens Gone Wild? Medical Anthropology and the 'Swine Flu' Pandemic." *Medical Anthropology* 28(3): 199–206.

Singer, Merrill, Freddie Valentin, Hans A. Baer, and Jia Zhongke. 1992. "Why Does Juan Garcia Have a Drinking Problem? The Perspective of Critical Medical Anthropology." *Medical Anthropology* 14(1): 77–108.

Smilde, David A. 1997. "The Fundamental Unity of the Conservative and Revolutionary Tendencies in Venezuelan Evangelicalism: The Case of Conjugal Relations." *Religion* 27(4): 343–359.

Smith, Daniel Jordan. 2004. "Youth, Sin and Sex in Nigeria: Christianity and HIV/AIDS." *Culture, Health, and Sexuality* 6(5): 425–437.

Smith, Daniel Jordan. 2014. *AIDS Doesn't Show Its Face: Inequality, Morality, and Social Change in Nigeria.* Chicago, IL: University of Chicago Press.

Smith, Linda Tuhiwai. 1999. *Decolonizing Methodologies: Researching and Indigenous Peoples.* London, United Kingdom: Zed Books Ltd.

Smith-Morris, Carolyn. 2006. *Diabetes among the Pima: Stories of Survival.* Tucson: University of Arizona Press.

Smith-Morris, Carolyn. 2007. "Autonomous Individuals or Self-Determined Communities? The Changing Ethics of Research among Native Americans." *Human Organization* 66(3): 327–336.

Snowdon, W., and A. M. Thow. 2013. "Trade Policy and Obesity Prevention: Challenges and Innovation in the Pacific Islands." *Obesity Reviews* 14(52): 150–158.

Sobal, J., and A. J. Stunkard. 1989. "Socioeconomic Status and Obesity: A Review of the Literature." *Psychological Bulletin* 105(2): 260–275.

Solomon, Harris. 2016. *Metabolic Living: Food, Fat, and the Absorption of Illness in India.* Durham, NC: Duke University Press.

Stearns, Peter. 2002. *Fat History: Bodies and Beauty in the Modern West.* New York, NY: New York University Press.

Stewart, William C., Michelle P. Adams, Jeanette A. Stewart, and Lindsay A. Nelson. 2013. "Review of Clinical Medicine and Religious Practice." *Journal of Religion and Health* 52(1): 91–106.

Strauss, Anselm L. 1984. *Chronic Illness and the Quality of Life.* Second Edition. St. Louis, MO: Mosby.

Stromberg, Peter. 1993. *Language and Self-Transformation: A Study of the Christian Conversion Narrative.* Cambridge, United Kingdom: Cambridge University Press.

Stunkard, A. J., and T. I. Sørensen. 1993. "Obesity and Socioeconomic Status—a Complex Relation." *The New England Journal of Medicine* 329(14): 1036–1037.

Suaalii-Sauni, Tamasailau M., Maualaivao Albert Wendt, Vitolia Mo'a, Naomi Fuamatu, Upolu Luma Va'ai, Reina Whaitiri, and Stephen L. Filipo. 2014. *Whispers and Vanities: Samoan Indigenous Knowledge and Religion.* Wellington, New Zealand: Huia Publishers.

Swanson, Anna. 2015. "The U.S. Isn't the Fattest Country in the World—But It's Close." *Washington Post.* www.washingtonpost.com/news/wonk/wp/2015/04/22/youll-never-guess-the-worlds-fattest-country-and-no-its-not-the-u-s/. Accessed May 23, 2016.

Swinburn, B. A., G. Sacks, K. D. Hall, K. McPherson, D. T. Finegood, M. L. Moodie, and S. L. Gortmaker. 2011. "The Global Obesity Pandemic: Shaped by Global Drivers and Local Environments." *The Lancet* 378: 804–814.

TallBear, Kim. 2014. "Standing with and Speaking as Faith: A Feminist-Indigenous Approach to Inquiry." *Journal of Research Practice* 10(2): 1–7.

Taylor, Janelle S. 2005. "Surfacing the Body Interior." *Annual Review of Anthropology* 34(1): 741–756.

Taylor, Janelle S. 2008. "On Recognition, Caring, and Dementia." *Medical Anthropology Quarterly* 22(4): 313–335.

Taylor, Nicole. 2015. *Schooled on Fat: What Teens Tell Us about Gender, Body Image, and Obesity.* New York: Routledge.

Taylor, Nicole. 2017. "Fat Is a Linguistic Issue: Discursive Negotiation of Power, Identity, and the Gendered Body among Youth." In *Fat Planet: Obesity, Culture and Symbolic Body Capital.* Eileen Anderson-Fye and Alexandra Brewis, eds. Pp. 125–148. Albuquerque: University of New Mexico Press.

Tcherkezoff, Serge. 2003. "A Long and Unfortunate Voyage Towards the 'Invention' of the Melanesia/Polynesia Distinction 1595–1832." Translated from French by Isabel Olivier. *The Journal of Pacific History* 38(2): 175–196.

Tengan, Ty Kawika. 2002. "(En)gendering Colonialism: Masculinities in Hawai'i and Aotearoa." *Cultural Values* 6(3): 239–256.

Tengan, Ty P. Kāwika. 2005. "Unsettling Ethnography: Tales of an 'Ō iwi in the Anthropological Slot." *Anthropological Forum* 15(3): 247–256.

Tengan, Ty P. Kāwika. 2008. *Native Men Remade: Gender and Nation in Contemporary Hawaii.* Durham, NC: Duke University Press.

Tengan, Ty P. Kāwika, and J. M. Markham. 2009. "Performing Polynesian Masculinities in American Football: From 'Rainbows to Warriors.'" *The International Journal of the History of Sport* 26(16): 2412–2431.

Tengan, Ty P. Kāwika, Tevita O. Ka'ili, and Rochlle Tuitagava'a Fonoti. 2010. "Genealogies: Articulating Indigenous Anthropology In/of Oceania." *Pacific Studies* 33(2/3): 139–167.

Thomas, Evert, Ina Vandebroek, Patrick Van Damme, Lucio Semo, and Zacarla Noza. 2009. "Susto Etiology and Treatment According to Bolivian Trintario People: A 'Masters of the Animal Species' Phenomenon." *Medical Anthropology Quarterly* 23(3): 298–319.

Thomas, Nicholas, Allen Abramson, Ivan Brady, R. C. Green, Marshall Sahlins, Rebecca A. Stephenson, Friedrich Valjavec, and Ralph Gardner White. 1989. "The Force of Ethnology: Origins and Significance of the Melanesia/Polynesia Division [and Comments and Replies]." *Current Anthropology* 30(1): 27–41.

Thornton, Alec, Tony Binns, and Maria Talaitupu Kerslake. 2013. "Hard Times in Apia? Urban Landlessness and the Church in Samoa: Urban Landlessness in Samoa." *Singapore Journal of Tropical Geography* 34(3): 357–372.

Thornton, Alec, Maria Kerslake, and Tony Binns. 2010. "Alienation and Obligation: Religion and Social Change in Samoa." *Asia Pacific Viewpoint* 51(1): 1–16.

Tomkins, Sandra M. 1992. "The Influenza Epidemic of 1918–19 in Western Samoa." *The Journal of Pacific History* 27(2): 181–197.

Trainer, Sarah, Alexandra Brewis, Daniel Hruschka, and Deborah Williams. 2015. "Translating Obesity: Navigating the Front Lines of the 'War on Fat.'" *American Journal of Human Biology* 27(1): 61–68.

Trainer, Sarah, Alexandra Brewis, Deborah Williams, and Jose Rosales Chavez. 2015. "Obese, Fat, or 'Just Big'? Young Adult Deployment of and Reactions to Weight Terms." *Human Organization* 74(3): 266–275.

Trainer, Sarah, Alexandra Brewis, Amber Wutich, Liza Kurtz, and Monet Niesluchowski. 2016. "The Fat Self in Virtual Communities: Success and Failure in Weight-Loss Blogging." *Current Anthropology* 57(4): 523–528.

Trnka, Susanna. 2017. *One Blue Child: Asthma, Responsibility, and the Politics of Global Health.* Stanford, CA: Stanford University Press.

Trnka, Susanna, and Catherine Trundle. 2014. "Competing Responsibilities: Moving Beyond Neoliberal Responsibilisation." *Anthropological Forum* 24(2): 136–153.

Trnka, Susanna, and Catherine Trundle. 2017. *Competing Responsibilities: The Ethics and Politics of Contemporary Life.* Durham, NC: Duke University Press.

Tuia, Tagataese Tupu, and Penelope Schoeffel. 2016. "Education and Culture in Post-colonial Sāmoa." *Journal of Samoan Studies* 6: 23–44.

Tuimaleaiʻfano, M. 2000. "Talof E Aiga: Ua ʻAi E Lago Le Tofa." In *Governance in Samoa: Pulega I Samoa*. E. Huffer and A. Soʻo, eds. Pp. 171–187. Palmerston North, New Zealand: Dunmore Press.

Tuimaleaiʻfano, M. 2006. "Matai Titles and Corruption in Modern Samoa: Costs, Expectations, and Consequences for Families and Society." In *Globalization and Governance in the Pacific Islands*, edited by Stewart Firth, 363–371. Canberra: Australian National University.

Tzioumis, Emma, and Linda S. Adair. 2014. "Childhood Dual Burden of Under- and Overnutrition in Low- and Middle-Income Countries: A Critical Review." *Food and Nutrition Bulletin* 35(2): 230–243.

Uchino, B. N. 2004. *Social Support and Physical Health: Understanding the Health Consequences of Relationships*. New Haven, CT: Yale University Press.

Ulijaszek, Stanley. 2005. "Modernisation, Migration and Nutritional Health of Pacific Island Populations." *Environmental Sciences: An International Journal of Environmental Physiology and Toxicology* 12(3): 167–176.

UN-OHRLLS. 2017. "Criteria for Identification of Graduate of LDCs." http://unohrlls.org/about-ldcs/criteria-for-ldcs/. Accessed May 2 2017.

United States State Department. 2003. *International Religious Freedom Report 2003: Samoa*. Washington, DC: Bureau of Democracy, Human Rights and Labor, U.S. Department of State.

Uperesa, Faʻanofo Lisaclaire. 2010. "A Different Weight: Tension and Promise in Indigenous Anthropology." *Pacific Studies* 33(2/3): 280–300.

Uperesa, Faʻanofo Lisaclaire. 2014. "Fabled Futures: Migration and Mobility for Samoans in American Football." *The Contemporary Pacific* 26(2): 281–301.

Uperesa, Faʻanofo Lisaclaire, and Tom Mountjoy. 2014. "Global Sport in the Pacific: A Brief Overview." *The Contemporary Pacific* 26(2): 263–279.

Vaʻai, Letuimanuʻasina Emma. 2012. "Religion." In *Samoa's Journey, 1962–2012: Aspects of History*. Wellington, New Zealand: Victoria University Press.

Vaʻa, Leulu Felise. 2001. *Saili Matagi: Samoan Migrants in Australia*. Suva, Fiji: Institute of Pacific Studies of the University of the South Pacific.

Valeri, Valerio. 1985. *Kingship and Sacrifice: Ritual and Society in Ancient Hawaii*. Chicago, IL: University of Chicago Press.

van Klinken, Adriaan. 2012. "Men in the Remaking: Conversion Narratives and Born Again Masculinity in Zambia." *Journal of Religion in Africa* 42(3): 215–239.

van Klinken, Adriaan. 2016. *Transforming Masculinities in African Christianity: Gender Controversies in Times of AIDS*. New York, NY: Routledge.

Vaughan, Megan. 1991. *Curing Their Ills: Colonial Power and African Illness*. Stanford, CA: Stanford University Press.

Village Population. 2016. *City Population*. www.citypopulation.de/Samoa.html.

Wang, Dongqing, Nicola L. Hawley, Avery A. Thompson, Viali Lameko, Muagatutia Sefuiva Reupena, Stephen T. McGarvey, and Ana Baylin. 2017. "Dietary Patterns Are Associated with Metabolic Outcomes among Adult Samoans in a Cross-Sectional Study." *The Journal of Nutrition* 147(4): 628–635.

Warren, Narelle, Rachel Canaway, Nalika Unantenne, and Lenore Manderson. 2013. "Taking Control: Complementary and Alternative Medicine in Diabetes and Cardiovascular Disease Management." *Health* 17(4): 323–339.

Weaver, Lesley Jo, and Craig Hadley. 2011. "Social Pathways in the Comorbidity between Type 2 Diabetes and Mental Health Concerns in a Pilot Study of Urban Middle- and Upper-Class Indian Women." *Ethos* 39(2): 211–225.

Weaver, Lesley Jo, and Emily Mendenhall. 2014. "Applying Syndemics and Chronicity: Interpretations from Studies of Poverty, Depression, and Diabetes." *Medical Anthropology* 33(2): 92–108.

Weiner, Annette B. 1992. *Inalienable Possessions: The Paradox of Keeping-While-Giving.* Berkeley: University of California Press.

Weller, S. C., R. D. Baer, L. M. Pachter, R. T. Trotter, M. Glazer, J. E. Garcia de Alba Garcia, and R. E. Klein. 1999. "Latino Beliefs about Diabetes." *Diabetes Care* 22(5): 722–728.

Weller, Susan C., Roberta D. Baer, Javier Garcia de Alba Garcia, and Ana L. Salcedo Rocha. 2008. "Susto and Nervios: Expressions for Stress and Depression." *Culture, Medicine, and Psychiatry* 32(3): 406–420.

Wells, Jonathan C. K., Akanksha A. Marphatia, Tim J. Cole, and David McCoy. 2012. "Associations of Economic and Gender Inequality with Global Obesity Prevalence: Understanding the Female Excess." *Social Science & Medicine* 75(3): 482–490.

Wendt, Albert. 1976. *Inside Us the Dead: Poems 1961 to 1974.* Auckland, New Zealand: Longman Paul.

Wendt, Albert. 1987. "Novelists and Historians and the Art of Remembering." In *Class and Culture in the South Pacific.* Anthony Hooper, ed. Pp. 78–91. Centre for Pacific Studies, University of Auckland, and Institute of Pacific Studies, University of the South Pacific.

West, Paige. 2005. "Holding the Story Forever: The Aesthetics of Ethnographic Labour." *Anthropological Forum* 15(3): 267–275.

West, Paige. 2016. "Teaching Decolonizing Methodologies." Savage Minds. July 25, 2016. https://savageminds.org/2016/07/25/teaching-decolonizing-methodologies/. Accessed May 21, 2018.

Whitehead, Harriet. 2000. *Food Rules: Hunting, Sharing, and Tabooing Game in Papua New Guinea.* Ann Arbor: University of Michigan Press.

Whitmarsh, Ian, and Elizabeth F. S. Roberts. 2016. "Nonsecular Medical Anthropology." *Medical Anthropology* 35(3): 203–208.

Whyte, Susan Reynolds. 2009. "Health Identities and Subjectivities: The Ethnographic Challenge." *Medical Anthropology Quarterly* 23(1): 6–15.

Whyte, Susan Reynolds. 2012. "Chronicity and Control: Framing the Ethnographic Challenge." *Anthropology and Medicine* 19(1): 63–74.

Wiedman, Dennis. 2012. "Native American Embodiment of the Chronicities of Modernity Reservation Food, Diabetes, and the Metabolic Syndrome among the Kiowa, Comanche, and Apache." *Medical Anthropology Quarterly* 26(4): 95–612.

Wiegele, K. 2005. *Investing in Miracles: El Shaddai and the Transformation of Popular Catholicism in the Philippines.* Honolulu: University of Hawaii Press.

Wilde, Charles. 2004. "Acts of Faith: Muscular Christianity and Masculinity among the Gogodala of Papua New Guinea." *Oceania* 75(1): 32–48.

Wilkinson, Richard, and Kate Pickett. 2010. *The Spirit Level: Why Equality Is Better for Everyone.* New York: Penguin Books.

World Council of Churches. N.d. Methodist Church of Samoa. www.oikoumene.org/en/member-Churches/methodist-Church-of-Samoa.

World Health Organization. "Preamble to the Constitution of WHO as Adopted by the International Health Conference." New York, 19 June–22 July 1946; signed on 22 July 1946 by the representatives of 61 states.

Yamamoto, M. 1994. "Urbanization of the Chiefly System: Multiplication and Role Differentiation of Titles in Western Samoa." *Journal of Polynesian Society* 103(2): 171–202.

Yates-Doerr, Emily. 2012a. "The Weight of the Self: Care and Compassion in Guatemalan Dietary Choices." *Medical Anthropology Quarterly* 26(1): 136–158.

Yates-Doerr, Emily. 2012b. "The Opacity of Reduction." *Food, Culture, and Society* 15(2): 293–313.

Yates-Doerr, Emily. 2013. "The Mismeasure of Obesity." In *Reconstructing Obesity Research: The Measures of Meaning, the Meaning of Measures.* Megan McCullough and Jessica Hardin, eds. Pp. 49–70. New York, NY: Berghahn Books.

Yates-Doerr, Emily. 2015. *The Weight of Obesity: Hunger and Global Health in Postwar Guatemala.* Berkeley, CA: University of California Press.

Yates-Doerr, Emily. 2016. "Fat Used to Be Celebrated in Guatemala, Now Unhelpful Obesity Advice Is Causing Weight Anxiety." The Conversation. http://theconversation.com/fat-used-to-be-celebrated-in-guatemala-now-unhelpful-obesity-advice-is-causing-weight-anxiety-67915. Accessed May 12, 2017.

Yates-Doerr, Emily, and Megan A. Carney. 2016. "Demedicalizing Health: The Kitchen as a Site of Care." *Medical Anthropology* 35(4): 305–321.

Young, Lani Wendt. 2013. "Your Sexual Abuse Is Disgusting and Has Brought Shame on Our Family." Sleepless in Samoa. https://laniwendtyoung.wordpress.com/2013/12/10/your-blog-is-disgusting-and-has-brought-shame-on-our-family/. Accessed August 5, 2017.

Young, Michael W. 1971. *Fighting with Food: Leadership, Values and Social Control in a Massim Society.* New York, NY: Cambridge University Press.

Zimmet, Paul. 1979. "Epidemiology of Diabetes and Its Macrovascular Manifestations in Pacific Populations: The Medical Effects of Social Progress." *Diabetes Care* 2:144–153.

Zimmet, Paul, K. G. Alberti, and J. Shaw. 2001. "Global and Societal Implications of the Diabetes Epidemic." *Nature* 414(6865): 782–787.

Zimmet, P., M. Arblaster, and K. Thoma. 1978. "The Effect of Westernization on Native Populations. Studies on a Micronesian Community with a High Diabetes Prevalence." *Australian and New Zealand Journal of Medicine* 8(2): 141–146.

Zimmet, P., G. Dowse, C. Finch, S. Serjeantson, and Hilary King. 1990. "The Epidemiology and Natural History of Niddm—Lessons from the South Pacific." *Diabetes/Metabolism Reviews* 6(2): 91–124.

Zola, Irving Kenneth. 1972. "Medicine as an Institution of Social Control." *The Sociological Review* 20(4): 487–504.

# INDEX

text messaging, 123; asking for assistance in, 130, 131–132, 133

thrifty gene, 47

tinned fish and meat, 33, 38, 45, 50, 52, 56, 57; gifts of, 67, 79; in supermarket aisle, 84

tithing, 92–93, 96, 99, 155n15

Tonga, life expectancy in, 47

*toto maualuga*, 2, 12, 73–74. *See also* high blood pressure

trade policies, 49, 82

traditional medicine and healers, 32, 108

*tulafale* (orators), 51, 54, 131, 160n4

Tupua Tamasese Mea'ole Hospital, 30

*umu* (earth oven), 38, 56

United States: fat talk in, 88, 99; medicalization of fat in, 10; migration to, 7, 48

*upu fa'aaloalo* (respect words), 155n15

Urapmin people, 159n12

urbanization, 42, 43, 48–49, 82; obesity in, 48, 53; physical activity in, 48, 49, 55

vegetables, 39, 57, 75, 121; cost of, 50, 58, 74, 116; in family plantations, 26, 27; as food gift, 84; in health promotion activities, 58–60; pesticides on, 45

VIDDA (violence, migration-related stress, depression, and domestic abuse), 46

voting rights, 51

wealth, 50–53; and body size, 12, 87, 90, 96, 99, 100; of congregation, church offerings in, 91; ethics of, 87, 94, 99, 100; and health, 12–13; institutional organization of, 20; of pastors, 13–14, 20, 52–53, 86, 90, 94, 96

weddings, 2, 51, 58, 92

weight, 4, 11; and body mass index, 10, 44, 47, 104, 154n12; and faith, 6; genetic factors in,

47; God as agent of change in, 119–120, 142; individual responsibility for, 10, 68–69, 76; joking and teasing comments about, 54; Know Your Numbers program on, 40; and medicalization of fat, 9–10; metric-centric approach to, 104; and obesity (*See* obesity); and self-hate feelings, 76; social context of, 40

well-being, 103–104; and faith, 119–121; God as source of, 142; and health, 104, 145, 159n2; in prayer, 105, 159–160n6

Wendt, Albert, 37, 85, 86

Western Samoa, 153n1

Williams, John, 156n1

*Witchcraft, Oracles, and Magic among the Azande* (Evans-Pritchard), 17

women: body size of, 76, 86; in church hierarchy, 125, 126; in community-based primary care, 31; as faletua (*See faletua*); and gendered suffering in Pentecostalism, 125, 155n19; on healing team, 105–111, 116, 123, 126, 136; mentoring relationships of, 80, 81, 98, 126, 130, 133, 137, 159n15; as nofotane, 158–159n10; obligations of, 128, 135; physical activity of, 54, 55; in prayer groups, 21, 98, 123–138; as prayer warriors, 126; puletasi of, 2, 122, 130; in radio ministry, 129; self-care of, 80, 81; self-evaluation of, 76, 128, 134; social and divine support of, 21, 123–138

worship, Christian, 4, 15, 22, 25–28, 40, 69, 73, 106, 117, 124, 126, 128, 133–134, 154n15, 159n13

World Bank, 43, 47

World Health Organization, 6, 43, 145

Young, Lani Wendt, 69, 70

Zumba, 55, 114, 115, 116

# ABOUT THE AUTHOR

JESSICA HARDIN is a medical anthropologist. She received her PhD from the Department of Anthropology at Brandeis University, where she also earned a joint MA degree in Anthropology and Women's and Gender Studies. She is an assistant professor at Pacific University, and she has also taught at the National University of Samoa. Her research and teaching interests span the fields of sociocultural anthropology, medical anthropology, feminist and women's studies, Pacific Studies, and the anthropology of Christianity. She is coeditor of the volume *Reconstructing Obesity: The Meaning of Measures and the Measure of Meanings*. Her work has been published in *Medical Anthropology; Medical Anthropology Quarterly; Food, Culture and Society; The Journal of Contemporary Religion; Anthropological Quarterly;* and *Critical Public Health*.